Ageing Well
Nutrition, Health, and Social Interventions

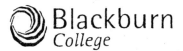

Society for the Study of Human Biology Series

10 Biological Aspects of Demography
Edited by W. Brass

11 Human Evolution
Edited by M. H. Day

12 Genetic Variation in Britain
Edited by D. F. Roberts and E. Sunderland

13 Human Variation and Natural Selection
Edited by D. Roberts (Penrose Memorial Volume reprint)

14 Chromosome Variation in Human Evolution
Edited by A. J. Boyce

15 Biology of Human Foetal Growth
Edited by D. F. Roberts

16 Human Ecology in the Tropics
Edited by J. P. Garlick and R. W. J. Keay

17 Physiological Variation and its Genetic Base
Edited by J. S. Weiner

18 Human Behaviour and Adaption
Edited by N. J. Blurton Jones and V. Reynolds

19 Demographic Patterns in Developed Societies
Edited by R. W. Hiorns

20 Disease and Urbanisation
Edited by E. J. Clegg and J. P. Garlick

21 Aspects of Human Evolution
Edited by C. B. Stringer

22 Energy and Effort
Edited by G. A. Harrison

23 Migration and Mobility
Edited by A. J. Boyce

24 Sexual Dimorphism
Edited by F. Newcome et al.

25 The Biology of Human Ageing
Edited by A. H. Bittles and K. J. Collins

26 Capacity for Work in the Tropics
Edited by K. J. Collins and D. F. Roberts

27 Genetic Variation and its Maintenance
Edited by D. F. Roberts and G. F. De Stefano

28 Human Mating Patterns
Edited by C. G. N. Mascie-Taylor and A. J. Boyce

29 The Physiology of Human Growth
Edited by J. M. Tanner and M. A. Preece

30 Diet and Disease
Edited by G. A. Harrison and J. Waterlow

31 Fertility and Resources
Edited by J. Landers and V. Reynolds

32 Urban Ecology and Health in the Third World
Edited by L. M. Schell, M. T. Smith and A. Billsborough

33 Isolation, Migration and Health
Edited by D. F. Roberts, N. Fujiki and K. Torizuka

34 Physical Activity and Health
Edited by N. G. Norgan

35 Seasonality and Human Ecology
Edited by S. J. Ulijaszek and S. S. Strickland

36 Body Composition Techniques in Health and Disease
Edited by P. S. W. Davies and T. J. Cole

37 Long-term Consequences of Early Environment
Edited by C. J. K. Henry and S. J. Ulijaszek

38 Molecular Biology and Human Diversity
Edited by A. J. Boyce and C. G. N. Mascie-Taylor

39 Human Biology and Social Inequality
Edited by S. S. Strickland and P. S. Shetty

40 Urbanism, Health and Human Biology in Industrialized Countries
Edited by L. M. Schell and S. J. Ulijaszek

41 Health and Ethnicity
Edited by H. Macbeth and P. S. Shetty

42 Human Biology and History
Edited by M. T. Smith

43 The Changing Face of Disease: Implications for Society
Edited by C. G. N. Mascie-Taylor, J. Peters and S. T. McGarvey

44 Childhood Obesity: Contemporary Issues
Edited by Noel Cameron, Nicholas G. Norgan, and George T. H. Ellison

45 The Nature of Difference: Science, Society and Human Biology
Edited by George T. H. Ellison and Alan H. Goodman

46 Social Information Transmission and Human Biology
Edited by Jonathan CK Wells, Simon Strickland, and Kevin Laland

47 Ageing Well: Nutrition, Health, and Social Interventions
Edited by Alan D. Dangour, Emily M. D. Grundy, and Astrid E. Fletcher

Numbers 1–9 were published by Pergamon Press, Headington Hill Hall, Headington, Oxford OX3 0BY. Numbers 10–24 were published by Taylor & Francis Ltd, 10–14 Macklin Street, London WC2B 5NF. Numbers 25–40 were published by Cambridge University Press, The Pitt Building, Trumpington Street Cambridge CB2 1RP. Further details and prices of back-list numbers are available from the Secretary of the Society for the Study of Human Biology.

Ageing Well
Nutrition, Health, and Social Interventions

Edited by
Alan D. Dangour, Emily M. D. Grundy, and Astrid E. Fletcher

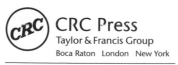

CRC Press
Taylor & Francis Group
Boca Raton London New York

CRC Press is an imprint of the
Taylor & Francis Group, an informa business

CRC Press
Taylor & Francis Group
6000 Broken Sound Parkway NW, Suite 300
Boca Raton, FL 33487-2742

Library of Congress Cataloging-in-Publication Data

Ageing well : nutrition, health, and social interventions / [edited by]
   Alan D. Dangour, Emily M. D. Grundy, Astrid E. Fletcher.
      p. ; cm. -- (Society for the Study of Human Biology ; 47)
   Includes bibliographical references and index.
   ISBN-13: 978-0-8493-7474-6 (hardcover : alk. paper)
   ISBN-10: 0-8493-7474-X (hardcover : alk. paper)
   1. Aging--Nutritional aspects. 2. Longevity--Social aspects. 3.
Aging--Prevention. I. Dangour, Alan D. II. Grundy, Emily M. D. III. Fletcher,
Astrid E. IV. Series: Society for the Study of Human Biology series ; 47.
   [DNLM: 1. Aging. 2. Developed Countries. 3. Health Policy. 4. Quality of Life.
5. Socioeconomic Factors. W1 SO861 v.47 2007 / WT 104 A2658 2007]

RA776.75.A344 2007
613.2--dc22   2006032432

Visit the Taylor & Francis Web site at
http://www.taylorandfrancis.com

and the CRC Press Web site at
http://www.crcpress.com

Dedication

This volume is dedicated to
Dr. Nicolas G. Norgan (1941–2006)
Chairman of the Society for the Study of Human Biology (2001–2005)

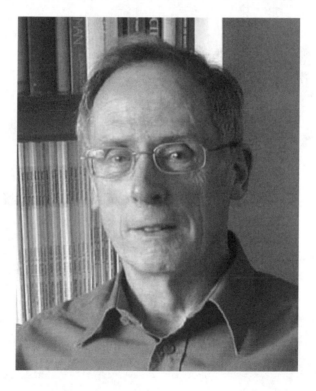

Contents

Chapter 1 Introduction 1
Alan D. Dangour, Emily M.D. Grundy, and Astrid F. Fletcher

Chapter 2 Nutritional concerns in old age.....................................5
Lisette C.P.G.M. de Groot and Wija A. van Staveren

Chapter 3 Regular exercise—the best investment for our old age 17
Marion E.T. McMurdo

**Chapter 4 Major eye diseases of later life: cataract and
age-related macular degeneration** 25
Astrid E. Fletcher

**Chapter 5 Reminiscence in everyday talk between older
people and their carers: implications for the quality of life
of older people in care homes**......................................35
*Fiona Wilson, Kevin McKee, Helen Elford, Man Cheung Chung,
Fiona Goudie, and Sharron Hinchliff*

**Chapter 6 Retention of cognitive function in old age:
why initial intelligence is important**.......................51
Lawrence J. Whalley

Chapter 7 Health inequalities in old age in Britain 67
Elizabeth Breeze

**Chapter 8 Demographic change, family support, and ageing well:
developed country perspectives**............................85
Emily M.D. Grundy

Chapter 9 Energy efficiency and the health of older people 103
Paul Wilkinson

Chapter 10   Ageing, health, and welfare: an economic perspective 117
Charles Normand

Chapter 11   Methodological issues in assessing the cost-effectiveness of interventions to improve the health of older people 127
Damian Walker and Cristian Aedo

Chapter 12   Minimum income for healthy living: older people in England, 2005–2006 139
*Jerry Morris, Alan D. Dangour, Christopher Deeming,
Astrid E. Fletcher, and Paul Wilkinson*

Chapter 13   Responding to increasing human longevity: policy, practice, and research 155
David Metz

Index 167

Editors

Alan D. Dangour is a lecturer in nutrition-related chronic disease at the London School of Hygiene & Tropical Medicine. Alan is a registered public health nutritionist, with a first degree in biochemistry, and postgraduate degrees in human nutrition and biological anthropology. Alan took up his current post at LSHTM in 2001 and, along with an active research portfolio, teaches extensively in the U.K. Nutrition Society-accredited Masters programme in public health nutrition. Alan has been a member of the Society for the Study of Human Biology committee since 1998 and was honorary secretary of the society from 2002 to 2005.

Alan's research focuses on public health nutrition interventions aimed at maintaining function and health in older age. Alan is the principal investigator of ongoing clinical trials funded by the U.K. Food Standards Agency examining the effect of supplementation with fish oil and vitamin B12 on cognitive and neurological function in older people in the United Kingdom. Alan also works on a large trial in Chile, funded by the Wellcome Trust, that aims to assess the cost-effectiveness of a national nutritional supplementation programme and an exercise intervention among older people in Santiago.

Emily M. D. Grundy is a professor of demographic gerontology at the London School of Hygiene & Tropical Medicine. Emily is a demographer and social gerontologist who has worked on aspects of individual and population ageing for over twenty years. Since 1998, she has worked in the Centre for Population Studies at LSHTM; previous appointments have been at the Institute of Gerontology, King's College London, and at City and Nottingham Universities.

Emily's main research interests are families, households and kin, and social networks in later life, especially in relationship to health, and trends and differentials in health, disability, and mortality at older ages. Currently, she is researching links between partnership and parenting histories and later life health. She is also involved in collaborative European projects on family support for older people and other collaborative projects in Latin America, mostly funded by the Economic and Social Research Council, the Nuffield Foundation, and the European Union. Emily is chair of the European Association for Population Working Group on Demographic Change and the Care of Older People, a member of the Census Advisory Committee, and on the editorial board of the *European Journal of Ageing*. Emily and colleagues from the Centre for Ageing and Public Health at LSHTM run an annual short course on ageing, health, and well-being in older populations.

Astrid E. Fletcher is a professor of epidemiology and ageing and director of the Centre for Ageing and Public Health, London School of Hygiene & Tropical Medicine. Astrid has a first degree in anthropology and postgraduate degrees in biological anthropology and epidemiology. She has held various research posts at the Institute of Cancer Research, University London College, and the Royal Postgraduate Medical School that focussed on cancer epidemiology, hypertension, and quality of life assessment. Astrid joined LSHTM in 1992 as senior lecturer and was promoted to professor in 1998.

Astrid has a portfolio of research in the epidemiology of ageing, including aetiology and evaluation of interventions and treatments. Most of her research is based in a U.K. and European context, and a substantial component is built around a large trial of community-based screening of older people in the United Kingdom, funded by the Medical Research Council and the Department of Health. Astrid's research on visual problems is primarily concerned with cataract and age-related macular degeneration. The now completed EU-funded EUREYE study assessed risk factors for macular degeneration in Europe, and an ongoing Wellcome Trust-funded study is assessing risk factors for cataract and macular degeneration among six thousand people aged over sixty years in India.

Contributors

Cristian Aedo
INACAP
Las Condes, Santiago, Chile

Elizabeth Breeze
Department of Epidemiology and
  Public Health
University College London
London, United Kingdom

Man Cheung Chung
School of Applied Psychosocial
  Studies
University of Plymouth
Plymouth, United Kingdom

Alan D. Dangour
Centre for Ageing and Public Health
London School of Hygiene &
  Tropical Medicine
London, United Kingdom

Christopher Deeming
School for Policy Studies
University of Bristol
Bristol, United Kingdom

Helen Elford
Sheffield Institute for Studies on
  Ageing
The University of Sheffield
Sheffield, United Kingdom

Astrid E. Fletcher
Centre for Ageing and Public Health
London School of Hygiene &
  Tropical Medicine
London, United Kingdom

Fiona Goudie
Community Health Sheffield
Sheffield, United Kingdom

Lisette C.P.G.M. de Groot
Department of Agrotechnology and
  Food Sciences
Division of Human Nutrition
Wageningen University
Wageningen, The Netherlands

Emily M. D. Grundy
Centre for Ageing and Public Health
London School of Hygiene &
  Tropical Medicine
London, United Kingdom

Sharron Hinchliff
Sheffield Institute for Studies on
  Ageing
The University of Sheffield
Sheffield, United Kingdom

Kevin McKee
Sheffield Institute for Studies on
  Ageing
The University of Sheffield
Sheffield, United Kingdom

Marion E. T. McMurdo
Division of Medicine and
  Therapeutics
University of Dundee
Dundee, United Kingdom

David Metz
Centre for Ageing and Public Health
London School of Hygiene &
  Tropical Medicine
London, United Kingdom

Jerry Morris
Public and Environmental Health
  Research Unit
London School of Hygiene &
  Tropical Medicine
London, United Kingdom

Charles Normand
Trinity College
University of Dublin
Dublin, Republic of Ireland

Wija A. van Staveren
Department of Agrotechnology and
  Food Sciences
Division of Human Nutrition
Wageningen University
Wageningen, The Netherlands

Damian Walker
Department of International
  Health
Bloomberg School of
  Public Health
Johns Hopkins University
Baltimore, Maryland, USA

Lawrence J. Whalley
Institute of Applied
  Health Sciences
University of Aberdeen
Aberdeen, United Kingdom

Paul Wilkinson
Centre for Ageing and
  Public Health
London School of Hygiene &
  Tropical Medicine
London, United Kingdom

Fiona Wilson
Sheffield Institute for Studies on
  Ageing
The University of Sheffield
Sheffield, United Kingdom

chapter one

Introduction

Alan D. Dangour, Emily M.D. Grundy, and Astrid E. Fletcher

Increased longevity in humans is one of the great biosocial and biomedical triumphs of the modern era. Globally, we are on average living longer and experiencing a better quality of life than ever before, although large differences between and within national populations remain. Increased longevity and generally declining fertility mean that all countries are experiencing growth in the numbers of older people in the population and, in many, the proportion of older people in the population is also expanding. By 2020 the world population of older people is expected to have trebled, with an estimated seven hundred million people aged sixty-five years and over, of whom 70% will be in developing countries. Of particular significance is the growth of the oldest old in the population.

Until recently, actions designed to have an impact on the health of older people have been limited. This has been due to a variety of factors, such as negative images of ageing, concepts that health promotion and disease prevention in old age are not worthwhile, and the research community's relative neglect of many of the common problems of old age. This lack of action is all the more surprising because the increase in the number of people living longer will have effects on many sectors of society. It is clear now that a multidisciplinary approach is required that fully integrates issues arising from population ageing and the needs of older people into all areas of public policy, including health, housing, economic development, and transport.

Many of the most important public health and policy concerns revolve around the apparent failing health of adults as they age. However, there is tremendous variation between individuals in the extent of age-related change and many changes once thought inevitable are now known to be capable of prevention, postponement, and, in some cases, reversal. This has led some to propose a clear distinction between usual and 'successful' ageing, or ageing well [1].

Recent work has shown that maintenance of healthy body weight, low cholesterol, low blood pressure, and regular physical activity results in significantly lower risk of incident dementia over a twenty-year follow-up amongst Finish older people [2]. Similarly, in a pan-European study, adherence to four simple healthy lifestyle characteristics—consumption of a Mediterranean style diet, moderate alcohol intake, regular physical activity, and not smoking—increased the chance of survival over ten years by more than 50% [3]. These kinds of regimes can be promoted by public health professionals and followed by individuals and do not depend on access to the best medical care or large financial resources.

For the forty-seventh annual symposium of the Society for the Study of Human Biology (SSHB), held in collaboration with the London School of Hygiene & Tropical Medicine Centre for Ageing and Public Health (CAPH) on 10 November 2005, experts from biomedical and biosocial backgrounds were invited to present state-of-the-art reviews on a range of health and social factors that affect the well-being of older people. The symposium, which was attended by academic researchers; health service personnel; members of governmental, nongovernmental, and older people's organisations; and interested members of the public, was designed to meet the joint aims of the SSHB and the CAPH. The objectives of the SSHB are the general advancement and promotion of research in the biology of human populations in all its branches, including human variability and genetics, human adaptability and ecology, and human evolution. The mission of the CAPH is to improve the health and well-being of older people in developed and developing countries.

This volume contains seven chapters written by speakers at the symposium, as well as five further chapters especially commissioned to broaden the book's scope. The aim of the volume is to highlight some of the important health and social factors affecting the well-being and quality of life of older people and to review possible interventions aimed at the prevention or amelioration of problems that reduce well-being and the potential for ageing well. The volume is not exhaustive in its coverage, but does discuss many of the everyday issues that affect the lives of older people, especially those living in developed countries.

In Chapter 2, Lisette de Groot and Wija van Staveren describe the extent of nutritional vulnerability in older people and highlight some of the major nutritional needs in later life. Promising results of nutritional and social interventions amongst frail older people demonstrate the benefit to health of a sufficient intake of a balanced diet provided in a good social environment. Marion McMurdo unequivocally emphasises the multiple benefits of regular exercise in older age in Chapter 3. Longitudinal studies frequently show moderate physical activity to be an important protective factor in later life, and international recommendations are uniform in their prescription of regular moderate-intensity physical activity. The deterioration of eye health with age and its impact on quality of life are discussed by Astrid Fletcher in Chapter 4. A review of observational and intervention research suggests that consumption of a diet rich in antioxidants and oily fish may be beneficial for eye health in later life.

Kevin McKee and colleagues consider the importance to older people of talking about past and present events in Chapter 5. The chapter highlights research showing that reminiscence provides an opportunity for development of a reciprocal, relationship-centred focus in care-giving settings that offers benefits in terms of social interaction and preservation of identity and well-being. In Chapter 6, Lawrence Whalley reviews findings from his extensive work on cognitive health in older age. Whilst the chapter shows that the level of initial intelligence is crucial in determining later life cognitive function, other factors, such as consumption of a healthy diet, judicious use of food supplements, not smoking, frequent health checks, and reduction of exposure to risk of vascular disease, are also essential for successful cognitive ageing.

The existence of significant health inequalities in older age is discussed in Chapter 7. Presenting data from two large studies of older people in the United Kingdom, Elizabeth Breeze highlights the presence of dramatic and insidious effects of socioeconomic status on a range of measures of health in older age. Chapter 8 provides an in-depth analysis of the importance of family support and kin networks in developed countries. Emily Grundy clearly demonstrates that trends in the demographic profiles of these countries will have positive outcomes in terms of provision of support in the short- to medium term, but that strong policy initiatives will be needed for the future. In Chapter 9, Paul Wilkinson highlights the effect of poor home environment, specifically indoor temperature, on mortality rates amongst older people in the United Kingdom. The rising cost of domestic fuel and the fact that many older people live in poor-quality houses make this a key policy issue for society to tackle.

Chapters 10 through 12 have an economic focus. First, in Chapter 10 the recurring concerns often aired in ageing societies, such as the cost of health care to national governments and the insufficiency of pension schemes, are discussed. Whilst there is no room for complacency, Charles Normand argues that, provided sensible policy decisions are taken, the future is not as bleak as is often forecast. The importance of assessing the cost-effectiveness of interventions aimed at improving the health of older people is highlighted in Chapter 11, which provides a general introduction to such analyses. Based on an ongoing study amongst older people (the CENEX Chile study), Damian Walker and Cristian Aedo also provide a useful example of the methodology for such studies. Finally, Chapter 12 brings together and provides costs of many of the needs of older people discussed in this volume. Jerry Morris and colleagues present their estimate of the minimum cost of healthy living for adults aged sixty-five years and older in the United Kingdom and compare it with the current level of state provision.

In the final chapter, David Metz discusses the many challenges to society and to the academic world resulting from increased longevity and urges more emphasis on ensuring good quality of life at the very end of life—a time in the life course when research is understandably very demanding to conduct. But this book is full of challenges, as is the future of all societies as they age. Are societies now ready to make the necessary changes and enact the needed policies? Time will tell, but inaction is surely not an option.

References

1. Rowe JW, Kahn RL. Human aging: Usual and successful. *Science* 1987, 237(4811):143–149.
2. Kivipelto M, Ngandu T, Laatikainen T, Winblad B, Soininen H, Tuomilehto J. Risk score for the prediction of dementia risk in 20 years among middle-aged people: A longitudinal, population-based study. *Lancet Neurol* 2006, 5(9):735–741.
3. Knoops KT, de Groot LC, Kromhout D, Perrin AE, Moreiras-Varela O, Menotti A, van Staveren WA. Mediterranean diet, lifestyle factors, and 10-year mortality in elderly European men and women: The HALE project. *JAMA* 2004, 292(12):1433–1439.

chapter two

Nutritional concerns in old age

Lisette C.P.G.M. de Groot and W.A. van Staveren

Contents

Summary 5
Introduction 6
The SENECA and HALE studies 6
Dietary pattern, lifestyle, and mortality 8
Addressing nutritional concerns in apparently healthy older people 8
    Vitamin D 8
    Vitamin B_{12} 9
Energy balance and energy intake in older people 10
Improving nutrient intake in frail or institutionalised older people 10
Conclusion 11
References 11

Summary

Physiological changes associated with ageing may have an impact on nutrient requirements in later life. As part of a healthful lifestyle, adherence to a high-quality diet is important for survival even in old age. Sufficient food consumption should help to ensure adequate intakes of most essential nutrients, although there are some exceptions, including vitamins D and B_{12}. Emerging evidence suggests that improving the intake of these latter nutrients may have beneficial effects on health in older age. Furthermore, several nutrition-related methods can decrease the progressive weight loss that occurs amongst older adults who habitually consume low-energy diets. It is becoming clear that, in older age, dietary quality and quantity are important for the maintenance of health and function.

Introduction

Although the process of ageing starts at adolescence or early adulthood [1], survival to at least sixty years, half the maximum human survival age, is necessary to reach old age. In the year 2000, 10% of the global population was aged sixty years or older, and this proportion is projected to reach 21% by 2050. Those surviving to sixty years of age can currently expect to live another seventeen (men) to twenty years (women) [2]. This extended life expectancy is not without cost, however, and results in an accumulation of cellular and molecular damage within the body [3]. When the various maintenance mechanisms in the body fail to preserve the normal structure of cells and tissues [4], a decline in many functions results and the risk of chronic diseases and impairments is likely to increase [5]. The pace of the accumulation of myriad tiny faults varies considerably between body systems, but eventually the viability of various organs is compromised [6].

This process is closely related to health status in older age, since the modification of lifestyle factors, including nutrition, appears to interact with ageing and health maintenance; the optimal outcome is the compression of morbidity and disability into a relatively short period before death [7]. Thus, in recent times, the focus on nutrition in older age has expanded from the prevention of macro- or micronutrient undernutrition to the critical role of diet in healthy ageing [8].

It has been argued from the public health perspective that food- (rather than nutrient-) based dietary approaches are the preferred way to address key nutritional issues amongst older people. Food-based dietary guidelines go beyond nutrients and food groups and include guidance on the way foods are produced, prepared, processed, and developed. Nutritional factors in such guidelines not only include dietary patterns but also address specific nutritional concerns relevant to older people [9]. Guidelines for older people emphasise the need to eat frequent small meals containing a good diversity of foods; to enjoy mealtimes, preferably eating in company; and to ensure adequate fluid intake. Guidance is also given, amongst other things, on the need to consume a healthy diet including good quantities of fruit and vegetables and two to three portions of fish (at least one portion of which should be oily) every week.

The SENECA and HALE studies

Nutritional deficiencies are more common at older ages than at other times in life. This is despite the fact that many older people eat well, but may be related to the fact that dietary variation between individuals is large in comparison to the variation found within individuals [10]. In the European setting, differences in social, cultural, and societal factors between countries were hypothesised to result in variations in markers of lifestyle and health outcomes [11]. In order to assess the importance of this diversity in diet and other lifestyle factors, the Survey in Europe on Nutrition and the Elderly: a Concerted Action (SENECA) was started in 1988 (*see* box).

The study was designed to assess regional and cross-cultural differences in nutrition, lifestyle, health, and performance of older Europeans and to explore the adequacy of diet in older age [12]. Selected survey towns were revisited five and ten years after the initial assessment in order to assess the impact of dietary and lifestyle variations on the ageing process and, in particular, on mortality risk. Similarities in design and data collection procedures allowed the merging of SENECA's data set with that of a comparable European prospective study (the Finland, Italy, the Netherlands Elderly [FINE] study) to become the HALE-project (Healthy Ageing: a Longitudinal Study in Europe) [13].

Design and methodology of SENECA

Approximately two thousand six hundred older people born between 1913 and 1918 living in nineteen 'traditional' towns in twelve countries were included. Site characteristics of the nineteen towns differed from rural to urban and from lowland to mountains, with a range of climates. The towns were selected to have stable populations of ten thousand to twenty thousand inhabitants and their population and economic structures were comparable to the average for each country. Participants were selected from an age- and sex-stratified sample of the inhabitants. Only people who were living in psychogeriatric nursing homes who were not fluent in the country's language or were not able to answer questions independently were excluded. The initial data collection in 1988–1989 was repeated with a follow-up in 1993 and a final data collection round in 1999. Full baseline and follow-up data were collected in the following towns: Hamme, Belgium; Roskilde, Denmark; Haguenau and Romans, France; Padua, Italy; Culemborg, the Netherlands; Vila Franca de Xira, Portugal; Betanzos, Spain; and Yverdon, Switzerland.

Data collection on lifestyle, morbidity, and mortality during the ten-year study was conducted using a standardised methodology across Europe and over time. For each town, equal numbers of men and women were selected. A nonresponder's questionnaire at baseline revealed that healthier and more health-concerned older people were more likely to participate in the study. In SENECA, the following items were assessed [59]:

- lifestyle, using a general structured interview questionnaire
- diet, using a modified dietary history consisting of a three-day record and a meal-based list of foods
- physical activities and activities of daily living
- smoking status

- nutritional status, by collecting anthropometrical and biochemical data
- health status and vital statistics

Dietary pattern, lifestyle, and mortality

Dietary pattern as a proxy for dietary quality has proved hard to quantify, and several different indices based on dietary guidelines have been developed. These indices or scores generally combine food groups and nutrients and rate diets based on the consumption of healthy and less healthy foods as defined by dietary guidelines [14]. Several longitudinal studies have demonstrated that these scores have an important predictive value [15,16].

Initial analysis of data from the SENECA study revealed that a lifestyle characterised by a high-quality diet, nonsmoking, and moderate physical activity contributes to healthy ageing: A healthy lifestyle was found to be positively related to a delay in the deterioration of health status [17] and to a decreased risk of death [18]. Subsequent data from the larger HALE study confirmed that amongst individuals aged seventy to ninety years, adherence to a Mediterranean type of diet pattern, moderate alcohol consumption, nonsmoking status, and moderate physical activity was each associated with a lower rate of all-cause mortality. Taken together, the combination was associated with a mortality rate of about one third that of those with none or only one of these four protective factors. These healthful behaviours did not need to be extreme; for example, the physical activity criterion could be met by as little as half an hour of walking daily [12]. These findings demonstrate that, even in older age, a simple set of healthy lifestyle practices appears to yield positive benefits for health and survival.

Addressing nutritional concerns in apparently healthy older people

Data from SENECA and other studies have suggested that average dietary intake levels of most nutrients are sufficient in older people [19]. However, vitamin D and vitamin B_{12}—low levels of which are often related to causes other than insufficient levels of dietary intake—are the exceptions.

Vitamin D

The requirement for dietary vitamin D depends on the amount of exposure to sunshine. In Europe about one third (about 4–5 µg/d) of total requirement for vitamin D (10–15 µg/d) originates from the diet. However, as a result of limited sunlight exposure and a fourfold reduced capacity of the skin to produce vitamin D with increasing age, deficiencies may occur in homebound older people [20]. Van der Wielen et al. [21] observed that 36% of men and 47% of women had serum hydroxyvitamin D values below 30 nmol/L (a frequently used cut-off for deficiency).

Counterintuitively, SENECA data showed that serum 25-hydroxyvitamin D concentrations were lowest amongst older people living in southern European countries [21]. Low concentrations were associated with negative attitudes to sunlight exposure and by higher levels of problems in performing activities of daily living in these populations. Both of these factors resulted in decreased exposure to sunlight and thus lower levels of endogenous vitamin D synthesis. However, regardless of geographic location, older people are at risk of having an inadequate vitamin D status in winter, and supplementation strategies should therefore be considered to improve bone health [22] and potentially also muscle function [23].

Given the high prevalence, severity, and health-care cost of osteoporotic fractures, cost-effective and well-tolerated prevention strategies are urgently needed. To achieve sufficient statistical power, intervention studies investigating the effect of vitamin D supplementation on fracture incidence require large numbers of study subjects and/or long follow-up periods [24]. To date, several randomised controlled trials have examined the effect of vitamin D supplements on the prevention of fracture in older people, but the results appear conflicting. Two secondary prevention studies in the United Kingdom did not support routine oral supplementation with calcium and vitamin D, either alone or in combination, for the prevention of further fractures in previously mobile elderly people [25] or in women with one or more risk factors for hip fracture [26]. However, a recent systematic review of available published literature that included a meta-analysis of randomised controlled trials suggested that oral vitamin D supplementation in the range of 700–800 IU/d should reduce the risk of hip or any nonvertebral fracture by approximately 25% [27]. A question to be addressed in future research is whether supplementation with calcium in addition to vitamin D enhances this apparently beneficial effect of vitamin D on fracture incidence.

Vitamin B_{12}

Low vitamin B_{12} (cobalamin) status is relatively common amongst older people and is partly a result of age-related gastric atrophy, which decreases the production of acid necessary for the release of B_{12} from the food matrix and results in B_{12} malabsorption. In contrast, crystalline B_{12} is well absorbed in most older people and oral supplementation and/or dietary fortification with crystalline B_{12} has been recommended to ensure adequate B_{12} status in later life.

In SENECA's follow-up study, van Asselt et al. [28] assessed vitamin B_{12} status in study participants and found mild deficiency to be present in 24% of the population. Interestingly, this deficiency could only partly be explained by inadequate cobalamin intake or severe atrophic gastritis. Usually, vitamin B_{12} deficiency is treated by monthly intramuscular injections of 1000 µg of hydroxycobalamin or cyanocobalamin. However, daily dietary supplementation with high oral doses of cyanocobalamin is considered as effective as intramuscular injections to correct biochemical markers of vitamin B_{12} deficiency. According to a recent dose-finding study, the amount of B_{12} required to correct certain metabolic abnormalities caused by B_{12} deficiency in older people is approximately two hundred times the recommended daily allowance for adults [29].

The metabolism of vitamin B_{12}, like that of several other B vitamins, is closely linked to that of homocysteine. The presence of high concentrations of homocysteine in blood indicates disrupted homocysteine metabolism, which has been linked to deficiencies of vitamin B_{12}, folate, and vitamin B_6 [30]. Raised levels of homocysteine appear to be associated to a range of detrimental health outcomes, such as the risk of atherosclerotic sequelae [31,32], the progression of cognitive decline [33], the development dementia and Alzheimer's disease [34], and even the incidence of fractures [35,36]. Such findings, which suggest that B vitamins can influence disease risk in older age, demonstrate the potential importance of adequate B vitamin status to promote optimal health. This is an exciting area of current research that requires some further support from efficacy studies [37,38].

Energy balance and energy intake in older people

Ageing is associated with an impairment in the regulation of food intake [39] and taste sensitivity [40]. The combined loss of homeostatic control and taste sensitivity has led to the development of the concept of physiologic anorexia of ageing, which has been defined as 'the physiological decrease in food intake occurring to counterbalance reduced physical activity and lower metabolic rate, not compensated in the long term' [41]. The existence of such a phenomenon has important implications for older people who for one reason or another may undergo a period of energy restriction. In the majority of these cases, such energy restriction will most likely result in a downward spiralling negative energy balance (i.e., progressive weight loss) [42]. The risk factors for low energy intake and progressive weight loss are especially prevalent in older people who become dependent. Importantly, decreases in energy turnover are associated not only with a decrease in energy intake but also with decreased intake of most other nutrients, which are typically ingested in proportion to energy. Thus, measures to counteract undernutrition in older people should be directed at increasing energy intake together with intake of other macronutrients, such as protein, and micronutrients.

Improving nutrient intake in frail or institutionalised older people

Older adults with low energy intakes must ensure that the foods that they consume have increased nutrient density. This translates into diets with increased concentrations of essential macro- and micronutrients, as opposed to low nutrient-density diets containing large amounts of refined sugars, fats, and alcohol. In a comparative study in the Netherlands, older women living in a nursing home had significantly lower energy intakes (6.5 ± 1.2 MJ/d) than physically active older women (8.8 ± 2.2 MJ/d) and even sedentary older women (7.7 ± 2.3 MJ/d) living at home. Even lower energy intakes were found amongst hospitalised women (6.0 ± 0.9 MJ/d) [43]. At the same time, no major differences in the selection of foods and dietary patterns emerged between community-dwelling older people and those dependent upon care [44]. Thus, once malnutrition or the risk of malnutrition presents itself, due attention should be given to sufficient food intake or early vigorous treatment of malnutrition.

Nutrient intake can be enhanced amongst older people by improving the quantity and/or the quality of dietary intake. Dietary intake quantity may be increased by improving access to food, providing feeding assistance [45], enhancing meal ambience [46,47], strengthening the flavour of food [48,49], and increasing energy demand via physical activity [50]. The quality of dietary intake may be improved by dietetic counselling, provision of nutrient-dense foods, and nutritional supplementation.

The effect of nutritional supplementation on biochemical indicators of nutritional status has been confirmed in a number of studies. According to a Cochrane Review by Milne et al. [51], supplementation produces a small but consistent weight gain in older people and a significant reduction in mortality risk (RR 0.74; 95% CI 0.59–0.92). There is currently limited evidence to suggest that nutritional supplementation can provide any functional benefits, but a few studies are beginning to provide suggestive evidence of benefit on outcomes related to physical and cognitive function [52–58].

Conclusion

In conclusion, physiological changes that occur with ageing have an impact, particularly on vitamin D and vitamin B_{12} needs. Diet may contribute to the provision of these nutrients but additional supplementation or the use of fortified foods may be needed. When energy intake of older people declines to levels below requirements, there are several ways to improve nutritional status, particularly of older people in care.

References

1. Bowling A, Ebrahim S. Glossaries in public health. *J Epidemiol Community Health*, 33, 223–226, 2001.
2. United Nations Population Division *World Population prospects*. The 2000 revision. www.un.org/esa/population/unpop.htm, 2001.
3. Kirkwood TBL. Evolution of aging. *Mechanisms Ageing Dev*, 123, 737–745, 2002.
4. Holliday R. Understanding ageing. *Phil Trans R Soc Lon B Biol Sci*, 352, 1793–1797, 1997.

5. Khaw KT. Epidemiologic aspects of ageing. *Phil Trans R Soc Lon B Biol Sci*, 52, 1829–1835, 1997.
6. Kirkwood TBL. Where will it all end? *Lancet*, 357, 567, 2001.
7. Campion EW. Aging better. *N Engl J Med*, 338(15), 1064–1066, 1998.
8. Rosenberg IH. Nutrition and aging. In: *Principles of Geriatric Medicine and Gerontology* (3rd ed.), ed. WR Hazzard, EL Bierman, JP Blass, WH Ettinger, JB Halter, R Andres. New York, McGraw–Hill, Inc, 49–60, 1994.
9. Wahlqvist ML. Malnutrition in the aged: The dietary assessment. *Public Health Nutr*, 5(6A), 911–913, 2002.
10. Van Staveren WA, de Groot LCPGM, Haveman-Nies A. The SENECA study: Potentials and problems in relating diet to survival over 10 years. *Public Health Nutr*, 5, 901–905, 2002.
11. de Groot LCPGM, van Staveren WA. SENECA's accomplishments and challenges. *Nutrition*, 16, 541–543, 2000.
12. van 't Hof MA, Hautvast JGAJ, Schroll M, Vlachonikolis IG. SENECA. Design, methods and participation. *Eur J Clin Nutr*, 45(suppl 3), 5–22, 1991.
13. Knoops KTB, de Groot LCPGM, Kromhout D et al. Mediterranean diet, life-style factors, and 10-year mortality in elderly European men and women. The HALE project. *JAMA*, 292, 1433–1439, 2004.
14. Jacques PF, Tucker KL. Are dietary patterns useful for understanding the role of diet in chronic disease? *Am J Clin Nutr*, 73, 1–2, 2001.
15. Trichopoulou A, Kouris-Blazos A, Wahlqvist ML, Gnardellis C, Lagiou P, Polychronopoulos E, Vassilakou T, Lipworth L, Trichopoulos D. Diet and overall survival in elderly people. *BMJ*, 311(7018), 1457–1460, 1995.
16. Trichopoulou A, Costacou T, Bamia C, Trichopoulos D. Adherence to a Mediterranean diet and survival in a Greek population. *N Engl J Med*, 348, 2599–2608, 2003.
17. Haveman-Nies A, de Groot LCPGM, van Staveren WA. Relation of dietary quality, physical activity and smoking habits to 10-year changes in health status in older Europeans in the SENECA study. *Am J Public Health*, 93, 318–323, 2003.
18. Haveman-Nies, de Groot CPGM, Burema J, Amorim Cruz, Osler M, van Staveren WA. Dietary quality and lifestyle factors in relation to 10-year mortality in elderly Europeans—The SENECA study. *Am J Epidemiol*, 156, 62–68, 2002.
19. de Groot CPGM, van den Broek T, van Staveren WA. Energy intake and micronutriënt intake in elderly Europeans. Seeking the minimum requirement in the SENECA study. *Age Ageing*, 28, 469–74, 1999.
20. Van Staveren WA. De Groot LCPGM. Vitamin D, nutritional significance. In: *Encyclopedia of Dairy Sciences*, ed. H Roginski, JW Fuquay, PF Fox. London, Academic Press, 2002.
21. van der Wielen RPJ, Lowik MRH, van den Berg H, de Groot LCPGM, Haller J, Moreiras O, van Staveren WA. Serum vitamin D concentrations among elderly people in Europe. *Lancet*, 346, 207–210, 1995.
22. Lips P. Vitamin D deficiency and secondary hyperparathryoidism in the elderly: Consequences for bone loss and fractures and therapeutic implications. *Endocrine Rev*, 22(4), 477–501, 2001.
23. Janssen HCJP, Samson MM, Verhaar HJJ. Vitamin D deficiency, muscle function, and falls in elderly people. *Am J Clin Nutr*, 75, 611–615, 2002.
24. Kanis JA. Treatment of osteoporotic fracture. *Lancet*, 1, 27–33, 1984.

25. The Record Trial Groups. Oral vitamin D3 and calcium for secondary prevention of low-trauma fractures in elderly people (randomised evaluation of calcium or vitamin D, RECORD): A randomised placebo-controlled trial. *Lancet*, 365, 1621–1628, 2005.
26. Porthouse J, Cockayne S, King C, et al. Randomised controlled trial of calcium and supplementation with cholecalciferol (vitamin D3) for prevention of fractures in primary care. *BMJ*, 330, 1003–1007, 2005.
27. Bischoff-Ferrari HA, Willett WC, Wong JB, Giovannucci E, Dietrich T, Dawson-Hughes B. Fracture prevention with vitamin D supplementation. *JAMA*, 293, 2257–2264, 2005.
28. van Asselt DZB, de Groot CPGM, van Staveren WA, et al. The role of cobalamin intake and atrophic gastritis in mild cobalamin deficiency in older Dutch subjects. *Am J Clin Nutr*, 68, 328–334, 1998.
29. Eussen SJPM, de Groot CPGM, Clarke R, Schneede J, Ueland PM, Hoefnagels WHL, van Staveren WA. Oral cyanocobalamin supplementation in older people with mild vitamin B12 deficiency. *Arch Intern Med*, 165, 1167–1172, 2005.
30. Selhub J, Bagley LC, Miller J, Rosenberg IH. B vitamins, homocysteine, and neurocognitive function in the elderly. *Am J Clin Nutr*, 71(2), 614S–620S, 2000.
31. Bots ML, Launer LJ, Lindemans J, Hofman A, Grobbee DE. Homocysteine, atherosclerosis and prevalent cardiovascular disease in the elderly: The Rotterdam Study. *J Intern Med*, 242, 339–347, 1997.
32. Bostom AG, Silbershatz H, Rosenberg IH, et al. Nonfasting plasma total homocysteine levels and all-cause and cardiovascular disease mortality in elderly Framingham men and women. *Arch Intern Med*, 159, 1077–1080, 1999.
33. Tucker KL, Qiao N, Scott T, Rosenberg I, Spiro A, III. High homocysteine and low B vitamins predict cognitive decline in aging men: The Veterans Affairs Normative Aging Study. *Am J Clin Nutr*, 82, 627–635, 2005.
34. Seshadri S, Beiser A, Selhub J, Jacques PF, Rosenberg IH, D'Agostino RB, Wilson PW, Wolf PA. Plasma homocysteine as a risk factor for dementia and Alzheimer's disease. *N Engl J Med*, 14, 346(7), 476–483, 2002.
35. McLean RR, Jacques PF, Selhub J, Tucker KL, Samelson EJ, Broe KE, Hannan MT, Cupples LA, Kiel DP. Homocysteine as a predictive factor for hip fracture in older persons. *N Engl J Med*, 350, 2042–2049, 2004.
36. Van Meurs JBJ, Dhonukshe-Rutten RAM, Pluijm SMF, et al. Homocysteine levels and the risk of osteoporotic fracture. *N Engl J Med*, 350, 2033–2041, 2004.
37. Malouf R, Areosa SA. Vitamin B12 for cognition. *Cochrane Database Systematic Rev*, 3, 2004.
38. van Asselt DZ, Pasman JW, van Lier HJ, Vingerhoets DM, Poels PJ, Kuin Y, Blom HJ, Hoefnagels WH. Cobalamin supplementation improves cognitive and cerebral function in older, cobalamin-deficient persons. *J Gerontol A Biol Sci Med Sci*, 56(12), M775–779, 2001.
39. Roberts SB, Fuss P, Heymann MB, et al. Control of food intake in older men. *JAMA*, 272, 1601–1606, 1994.
40. de Graaf C, Polet P, van Staveren WA. Sensory perception and pleasantness of food flavors in elderly subjects. *J Gerontol*, 49, P93–99, 1994.
41. Morley JE. Anorexia of aging: Physiologic and pathologic. *Am J Clin Nutr*, 66, 760–773, 1997.
42. Egbert AM. The dwindles: Failure to thrive in older patients. *Nutr Rev*, 54, S25–30, 1996.

43. de Groot CPGM, van Staveren WA, de Graaf C. Determinants of macronutri-
    ent intake in elderly people. *Eur J Clin Nutr*, 54, suppl 3, S70–76, 2000.
44. Van der Wielen RP, de Wild GM, de Groot LC, Hoefnagels WH, van Staveren
    WA. Dietary intakes of energy and water-soluble vitamins in different cate-
    gories of aging. *J Gerontol A Biol Sci Med Sci*, 51, B100–107, 1996.
45. Simmons SF, Osterweil D, Schnelle JF. Improving food intake in nursing home
    residents with feeding assistance: A staffing analysis. *J Gerontol A Biol Sci Med
    Sci*, 56(12), M790–794, 2001.
46. Mathey MF, Vanneste VG, de Graaf C, de Groot LC, van Staveren WA. Health
    effect of improved meal ambiance in a Dutch nursing home: A 1-year inter-
    vention study. *Prev Med*, 32(5), 416–423, 2001.
47. Nijs KA, de Graaf C, Kok FJ, van Staveren WA. Family style meals maintain
    the quality of life, physical performance and body weight of nursing home
    residents. *BMJ*, 332, 1180–1184, 2006.
48. Schiffman SS, Graham BG. Taste and smell perception affect appetite and
    immunity in the elderly. *Eur J Clin Nutr*, 54, suppl 3, S54–63, 2000.
49. Mathey MF, Siebelink E, de Graaf C, Van Staveren WA. Flavor enhancement
    of food improves dietary intake and nutritional status of elderly nursing home
    residents. *J Gerontol A Biol Sci Med Sci*, 56(4), M200–205, 2001.
50. Chin A, Paw MJ, de Jong N, Schouten EG, van Staveren WA, Kok FJ. Physical
    exercise or micronutrient supplementation for the well-being of the frail eld-
    erly? A randomised controlled trial. *Br J Sports Med*, 36(2), 26–31, 2002.
51. Milne AC, Potter J, Avenell A. Protein and energy supplementation in elderly
    people at risk from malnutrition. *Cochrane Database Systematic Rev, Issue 1, Art
    No. CD003288. DOI: 10.1002/146518858 CD003288, pub 2, 2005.
52. de Jong N, Chin A, Paw MJ, de Groot LC, Rutten RA, Swinkels DW, Kok FJ,
    van Staveren WA. Nutrient-dense foods and exercise in frail elderly: Effects
    on B vitamins, homocysteine, methylmalonic acid, and neuropsychological
    functioning. *Am J Clin Nutr*, 73(2), 338–346, 2001.
53. de Jong N, Chin A, Paw MJ, de Groot LC, Hiddink GJ, van Staveren WA.
    Dietary supplements and physical exercise affecting bone and body compo-
    sition in frail elderly persons. *Am J Public Health* 90(6), 947–954, 2000.
54. Manders M, de Groot CPGM, van Staveren WA, Wouters-Wesseling M, Mul-
    ders AJ, Schols JM, Hoefnagels WH. Effectiveness of nutritional supplements
    on cognitive functioning in elderly persons: A systematic review. *J Gerontol
    A Biol Sci Med Sci*, 59(10), 1041–1049, 2004.
55. Wouters-Wesseling W, Wouters AE, Kleijer CN, Bindels JG, de Groot CP, van
    Staveren WA. Study of the effect of a liquid nutrition supplement on the
    nutritional status of psychogeriatric nursing home patients. *Eur J Clin Nutr*,
    56(3), 245–251, 2002.
56. Wouters-Wesseling W, Vos AP, Van Hal M, De Groot LC, Van Staveren WA,
    Bindels JG. The effect of supplementation with an enriched drink on indices
    of immune function in frail elderly. *J Nutr Health Aging*, 9(4), 281–286, 2005.
57. Wouters-Wesseling W, Wagenaar LW, Rozendaal M, Deijen JB, de Groot LC,
    Bindels JG, van Staveren WA. Effect of an enriched drink on cognitive function
    in frail elderly persons. *J Gerontol A Biol Sci Med Sci*, 60(2), 265–270, 2005.
58. Wouters-Wesseling W, Van Hooijdonk C, Wagenaar L, Bindels J, de Groot L,
    Van Staveren W. The effect of a liquid nutrition supplement on body compo-
    sition and physical functioning in elderly people. *Clin Nutr*, 22(4), 371–377,
    2003.

59. de Groot CPGM, Verheijden MW, de Henauw S, Schroll M, van Staveren WA. Lifestyle, nutritional status, health and mortality in elderly people across Europe: A review of the longitudinal results of the SENECA study. *J Ger Med Sci*, 59A, 1277–1284, 2004.

chapter three

Regular exercise—the best investment for our old age

Marion E.T. McMurdo*

Contents

Introduction 17
Physical activity versus exercise 18
Determinants, barriers, and safety..19
Conclusion 21
References..22

Introduction

Although increasing life expectancy is hailed by some as one of the greatest achievements of the twentieth century, a more common reaction is a doom-laden prediction of health and social budgets being bled dry by the burden of caring for dependent old people. This overwhelmingly negative reaction has been fuelled by a misunderstanding about health in old age. Of course, we need to consider how best to care for our growing older population, but this aspect has dominated debate to the near exclusion of the development of strategies with the potential to increase disability-free later life. Future health and social care needs will be determined not by the absolute numbers of older people, but by what proportion of this number are disabled and require care. Certainly, older people often have poorer health than younger people, due in part to the higher rates of disease in old age. The incidence of heart disease, for example, increases with increasing

* Conflict of interest: METM is codirector of D. D. Developments Limited, a University of Dundee company, the mission of which is to provide exercise classes for older people throughout the United Kingdom. Any profits support ageing research.

age. This does not mean, however, that old age causes heart disease, nor does it mean that heart disease is an inevitable accompaniment of old age. Finally, laying to rest the myth that all the ills of old age are 'just your age' would represent a massive breakthrough for the health care of older people.

There are essentially five major influences on our experience of health and disease: genetic, environmental (social and economic), lifestyle, nutrition, and chance. The old adage to 'choose your parents well' is undoubtedly correct because long-lived parents tend to produce long-lived children. However, those who lack long-lived parents or grandparents may be comforted by the knowledge that only an estimated 25% of how long we live is genetically determined. Whilst poverty, poor housing, low incomes, and social isolation make a significant adverse contribution to health, solutions to such problems continue to elude most governments. Probably the most readily modifiable influences on health are lifestyle and nutrition. Although lifestyle issues should not be considered in complete isolation from each other, this chapter will focus on the influence of physical activity on health and disability in old age.

Physical activity versus exercise

Physical activity is different from exercise and the terms should not be used interchangeably. Physical activity is bodily movement produced by the contraction of skeletal muscle that increases energy expenditure. Intensity of physical activity is defined subjectively in metabolic equivalents (METs). One MET is the energy expenditure for sitting quietly, which for the average adult approximates 3.5 mL of oxygen uptake per kilogram of body weight per minute. A 3-MET activity therefore requires three times the metabolic energy expenditure of sitting quietly. Recommendations suggest that most adults should be participating in thirty minutes of moderate-intensity (3–6 METs) physical activity on most days of the week [1]. This dose is associated with most health benefits and does not require participation in formal exercise programmes. Moderate-intensity activities include brisk walking, cycling on the flat, dancing, golf wheeling or carrying clubs, recreational swimming, gardening, and moderate housework. For older people, classification of activity intensity might be higher; for example, what constitutes moderate-intensity activity for a forty-five-year-old may well represent vigorous-intensity activity for a seventy-five-year-old.

Exercise is a subset of physical activity and is defined as planned, structured, repetitive movement done with the express purpose of improving or maintaining physical fitness. Whilst most of the population indulges in some incidental physical activity during the course of the day, precious few of us are taking any exercise.

Whilst disability in old age is not just about loss of muscle strength, muscle weakness and low exercise levels present tantalisingly modifiable targets. A prospective cohort study in community-dwelling older women identified slow gait, short-acting benzodiazepine use, depression, low exercise levels, and obesity as significant modifiable predictors of decline [2]. Physical capacity peaks in young adulthood and then declines progressively decade by decade at a rate that varies from one individual to another. For a young person, lack of fitness will be apparent only if he is required to perform vigorous activity—for example, to play a game of football. He will, however, have ample reserves to cope with the demands of daily life, climb stairs, go to the shops, and socialise with friends. This is in stark contrast to the older person who may be precariously close to the threshold where a small decline in fitness will render everyday activities, like rising from an armchair, impossible.

Part of this physical decline is due to ageing and is not amenable to intervention. Even healthy ageing is associated with a striking loss of muscle mass and hence muscle strength; by the age of eighty years, approximately 50% of our youthful muscle mass has gone. However, it is now appreciated that some age-related changes that were once accepted to be solely the result of the ageing process are actually the result of muscle disuse and therefore potentially reversible. The small added loss of fitness that occurs in association with an episode of intercurrent illness may render even a previously healthy eighty-year-old immobile and dependent. However, there is substantial evidence that lost fitness can be regained with regular physical activity, even in extreme old age. The trainability of muscles of even very old people has been demonstrated, [3] with one study reporting a 15.5% increase in maximal voluntary contraction of the quadriceps muscle in response to a six-month programme of seated exercise in very old residents of old people's homes [4]. Whilst it is encouraging that old muscles are trainable, this observation is important only if having stronger muscles actually makes daily life easier to accomplish.

Strength training does not halt the underlying loss of muscle fibres, but the improvements in strength reported in studies of exercise training in older people may be equivalent to ten to twenty years of 'rejuvenation' and may prevent an individual from falling beneath functionally important thresholds [5,6]. For functionally impaired older women, walking as little as eight blocks per week was associated with better health and function than that seen in nonwalkers [7]. Although this is an exceedingly modest amount of activity by public health standards, it was sufficient in this particular cohort; the greatest benefits were found in the subset with the most severe limitations. If such disability-delaying effects were insufficiently compelling in themselves, then there is also evidence that participation in regular physical activity is protective against a range of diseases, including heart disease, diabetes, some cancers, osteoporosis, mild depression, and Alzheimer's disease and dementia [8].

Determinants, barriers, and safety

Demonstrating that exercise can be beneficial is considerably less difficult than persuading people to be more physically active. The Scottish Health

Survey has revealed a woefully inactive population with a disappointingly low proportion reporting participation in recommended levels of physical activity (i.e., thirty minutes of moderate-intensity physical activity on most days of the week). Given that the survey is based on self-report, cynics may suspect that actual participation levels might be even lower. A study in Canada found that many of the population were so unfit that walking at three miles per hour up an incline involved severe exertion [9]. It is easy to see why so many are discouraged before they begin.

Many older people participate in no leisure time activity at all [10], despite generally high levels of knowledge about the specific benefits of physical activity. A study of 409 randomly selected community-dwelling older people found that almost all participants believed that physical activity was beneficial, and 79% believed that they did enough to keep healthy. However, 36% did no leisure time activity and a further 17% did less than two hours per week. The most powerful deterrents were lack of interest (odds ratio = 7.8), lack of access to a car, shortness of breath, joint pain, dislike of going out alone, perceived lack of fitness, doubting that exercise can lengthen life, not belonging to a group, and doubting that meeting new people is beneficial [11].

Part of the problem is the common misconception that to reap health benefits, continuous, vigorous exercise (athletics, jogging, or squash) is required. This notion has its origins in studies of the effects of endurance exercise training on maximal oxygen uptake in younger adults. This work produced a physical fitness recommendation of twenty to sixty minutes of endurance exercise at 60–90% of maximal heart rate, three or more times per week. This advice was so scientific, complex, and prescriptive and set such an unattainable goal for sedentary and older people that many must have given up on exercise as a lost cause. However, a reassessment of the original evidence together with a growing body of new research has shown that the majority of health benefits can be gained by performing regular moderate-intensity physical activities (the equivalent of brisk walking at three to four miles per hour for most healthy adults) [1].

This good news for couch potatoes of all ages is particularly heartening for older people who find it is much easier to adopt and maintain more modest activity levels. It carries the added bonus that low- to moderate-intensity physical activities are more likely to be continued than high-intensity activities. Determinants of participation in exercise or physical activity include enjoyment; confidence in the ability/safety to be active; goal setting; and encouragement from significant others, including family, friends, neighbours, and health-care workers.

Safety is a key consideration when promoting physical activity and exercise for older people, although the risks are frequently overestimated, particularly in the minds of the medical profession. Inactivity in old age is reinforced by stereotypical views on the inevitability of decline with ageing and on a lack of understanding of the trainability of even very ancient muscles. This may be worsened by well-intentioned relatives taking over the household chores, inadvertently depriving their older relative of his or her main physical activity of the week.

Older people are often less ambitious exercisers, so traumatic and over-use injuries are less common in middle-aged people preparing for competitions than in their younger counterparts. Factors likely to contribute to a high injury rates are failure to warm up adequately; violent exercises, especially twisting movements; too rapid progression of training with exercise continuing beyond the point of pleasant fatigue; exercise on a hard or uneven surface; and the use of shoes with inadequate heels and poor ankle support. Warning symptoms include undue breathlessness, chest pain, or dizziness. However, if activity is not provoking symptoms, it is very unlikely to be doing harm.

Probably the single most damaging phrase that has come to be associated with exercise in recent years is 'no pain, no gain'. This dangerous axiom exhorts a mindless, competitive edge and is the cause of innumerable injuries to people of all ages. It has no place in a strategy of pleasurable, lifelong physical activity. No older person should be discouraged from becoming more physically active as immobility and a sedentary state are harbingers of morbidity and mortality. People returning to activity after a gap of many years should be encouraged to start slowly, build up gradually, and always remain within their individual levels of comfort.

Conclusion

It is unfortunate that public health advice has failed to shake off the 'high-tech', lycra-clad image of aerobic exercise and physical fitness and embrace the broader concept of health and physical activity—walking, dancing, bowling, or gardening. The sedentary state has become so all pervasive that we have lost sight of the fact that physical activity is part of normal, reasonable, health-enhancing behaviour across the age spectrum [12]. Modern man remains adapted for the life of a hunter–gatherer, with food in scarce supply and obtained only after strenuous, and frequently unsuccessful, hunts. In contrast to this, food is taken for granted in the developed world, available twenty-four hours a day, and energy expenditure per kilogram is estimated at only 38% of our Palaeolithic ancestors [13]. Western societies are already reaping the harvest of a sedentary lifestyle with which we are ill equipped to deal, with alarming increases in rates of obesity and diabetes. Compelling evidence exists of the benefits of regular physical activity in old age, and older people who need information about how to preserve their health should be listened 'to' before they are talked 'at'. Regrettably, many clinicians lack the skills, knowledge, inclination, and reimbursement to discuss physical activity routinely with their older patients, although this has been shown to be effective [14]. The message should be that doing some regular physical activity is better than doing none and that doing exercise is even better.

If the older community in general is to benefit from a more active lifestyle, then a rehabilitative approach must be adopted by community services. Current systems are overly ready to *do everything* for older people who are struggling with mobility or self-care and far too uncritical in thinking about *why* an older person now needs assistance. Rapid access to specialist assessment and investigation is essential for the proper care of older people in whom illness may present in a muted or atypical fashion and so pass unrecognised until the window of opportunity for successful treatment may have closed forever. Older people must be informed that regular physical activity is appropriate and desirable in old age, and the older community should be engaged to develop services and facilities to back this up. It is time to challenge the notion that old age is the time to slow down, hang up your boots, and sit in an armchair by taking a positive stance to promote physical activity for older people.

References

1. Pate RR, Pratt M, Blair SN, Haskell WL, Macera CA, Bouchard C, Buchner D, Ettinger W, Heath GW, King AC et al. Physical activity and public health. A recommendation from the Centers for Disease Control and Prevention and the American College of Sports Medicine. *JAMA* 1995, 273(5):402–407.
2. Sarkisian CA, Liu H, Gutierrez PR, Seeley DG, Cummings SR, Mangione CM. Modifiable risk factors predict functional decline among older women: A prospectively validated clinical prediction tool. The Study of Osteoporotic Fractures Research Group. *J Am Geriatr Soc* 2000, 48(2):170–178.
3. Fiatarone MA, Marks EC, Ryan ND, Meredith CN, Lipsitz LA, Evans WJ. High-intensity strength training in nonagenarians. Effects on skeletal muscle. *JAMA* 1990, 263(22):3029–3034.
4. McMurdo ME, Rennie LM. Improvements in quadriceps strength with regular seated exercise in the institutionalized elderly. *Arch Phys Med Rehabil* 1994, 75(5):600–603.
5. Malbut-Shennan K, Young A. The physiology of physical performance and training in old age. *Coronary Artery Dis* 1999, 10(1):37–42.
6. McMurdo ME, Rennie L. A controlled trial of exercise by residents of old people's homes. *Age Ageing* 1993, 22(1):11–15.
7. Simonsick EM, Guralnik JM, Volpato S, Balfour J, Fried LP. Just get out the door! Importance of walking outside the home for maintaining mobility: Findings from the Women's Health and Aging Study. *J Am Geriatr Soc* 2005, 53(2):198–203.
8. Rovio S, Kareholt I, Helkala EL, Viitanen M, Winblad B, Tuomilehto J, Soininen H, Nissinen A, Kivipelto M. Leisure-time physical activity at midlife and the risk of dementia and Alzheimer's disease. *Lancet Neurol* 2005, 4(11):705–711.
9. Stephens T, Craig CL, Ferris BF. Adult physical activity in Canada: Findings from the Canada Fitness Survey I. *Can J Public Health* 1986, 77(4):285–290.
10. Yusuf HR, Croft JB, Giles WH, Anda RF, Casper ML, Caspersen CJ, Jones DA. Leisure-time physical activity among older adults. United States, 1990. *Arch Intern Med* 1996, 156(12):1321–1326.

11. Crombie IK, Irvine L, Williams B, McGinnis AR, Slane PW, Alder EM, McMurdo ME. Why older people do not participate in leisure time physical activity: A survey of activity levels, beliefs and deterrents. *Age Ageing* 2004, 33(3):287–292.
12. McMurdo ME. Exercise in old age: Time to unwrap the cotton wool. *Br J Sports Med* 1999, 33(5):295–296.
13. Hambrecht R, Gielen S. Essay: Hunter–gatherer to sedentary lifestyle. *Lancet* 2005, 366, suppl 1:S60–61.
14. Calfas KJ, Long BJ, Sallis JF, Wooten WJ, Pratt M, Patrick K. A controlled trial of physician counseling to promote the adoption of physical activity. *Prev Med* 1996, 25(3):225–233.

chapter four

Major eye diseases of later life: cataract and age-related macular degeneration

Astrid E. Fletcher

Contents

Vision impairment in later life 25
    Cataract..26
    Age-related macular degeneration (AMD)................................26
Factors that may increase the risk of cataract or AMD 27
    Smoking..27
    Light exposure...27
    Genetic susceptibility 28
    Dietary factors 28
        Antioxidants..28
        Dietary fat..30
Conclusions..31
References..31

Vision impairment in later life

It is well known that vision deteriorates in old age. Distance visual acuity (VA) is reduced and problems with near vision activities, such as reading, increase. Studies in high-income countries such as the United Kingdom and United States show that the prevalence of visual impairment, measured by distance acuity, rises from around the age of sixty years. Using a criterion of VA < 6/12 (equivalent to the visual standard required for driving in most countries) around one in one hundred people is impaired at ages sixty to sixty-four, rising to nearly one in five at age eighty and above [1]. The major causes of visual impairment in the older population are refractive errors, cataracts, and age-related macular degeneration (AMD) [1,2]. Diabetic retinopathy and glaucoma account for less than 10% of vision impairment in the older population in the United Kingdom [2], but for a higher proportion of blindness due to their progressive nature. Refractive errors are due to problems with accommodation (light focussing on the back of the eye) and are corrected by spectacles or contact lenses.

Cataract

Cataract is dense opacification of the lens interfering with vision and can be treated by removal of the lens and replacement with a plastic lens. Lens opacification arises in a number of ways, principally increasing insolubility and unfolding of the crystalline protein of the lens fibres leading to disruption of the refractive index, light scattering, and loss of transparency. As a result, glare, especially at night, is one of the first symptoms noticed by people. With increasing opacification, the vision becomes blurred. Cataracts or lens opacities are also described according to their anatomical position in the lens—that is, nuclear (centre) or cortical (outer region). Posterior subcapsular opacities (PSCs), which occur at the back of the lens and under the lens capsule, cause greater interference with vision because they lie more directly in the line of vision. Although it is asserted that different types of opacities may have different risk factors, the evidence is limited by the fact that most opacities in older people are mixed. The lens has no blood supply and nutrients and waste products are obtained from the surrounding aqueous fluid through the lens capsule.

Age-related macular degeneration (AMD)

AMD is a condition characterised by loss of central vision due to damage to the macular region of the retina; it is the major cause of blindness registration in high-income countries. AMD is rare in middle and early old age. The highest prevalence is observed in the oldest age group: Around one in ten people over the age of eighty years has AMD. There are two main types of AMD. Neovascular AMD (NVAMD, or 'wet' AMD) is characterised by growth and invasion of new blood vessels often leaking blood and fluid. Geographic atrophy (GA, or 'dry' AMD) is characterised by extensive loss of the layer of capillaries adjacent to the retina and the overlying retinal pigment epithelium (RPE). In most populations of European origin, the prevalence of NVAMD is around twofold that of GA. Whilst vision loss in both can be extensive, NVAMD accounts for 90% of all subjects registered as blind due to AMD. Although some improvements have been made in the treatment of AMD, at best they slow the rate of vision loss in a minority of patients.

Many people in the older population will have morphological changes in the retina including drusen (small yellowish deposits) and irregularities in the RPE. Collectively, these changes are known as early age-related maculopathy, or ARM, with increasing severity of ARM characterised by larger soft drusen and greater RPE irregularities. There has been intense debate as to whether these changes represent the earliest manifestations of AMD. Longitudinal studies of population-based cohorts show that certain types of drusen (hard drusen) are not predictive of progression to AMD, but that those with more severe features have a higher risk. For example, the five-year risk of incident AMD in the Rotterdam study was around 1%. However, for those with large soft indistinct drusen or pigmentary abnormalities at baseline, the five-year risk of incident AMD was 28%, ranging from 17.5% in those aged sixty to sixty-nine at baseline to 42% for those aged eighty and over [3].

Factors that may increase the risk of cataract or AMD

Smoking

Smoking has been consistently identified as a risk factor for cataract and AMD [4,5]. That the association is likely to be causal is suggested by the consistency of the association across different study designs and populations, a dose–response relationship, and a reduction in risk with length of smoking cessation.

Light exposure

The eye is, of necessity, particularly vulnerable to the adverse effects of light exposure. The lens, along with the cornea, plays a vital role in reducing the harmful effects of solar radiation by absorption of the shorter wavelengths of light in the range known as ultraviolet radiation (UVR). The pathways through which UVR adversely damages the lens are not well understood but include generation of reactive oxygen species (ROS) resulting in protein modification. The lens also transmits and focuses visible light to the retina. Thus, the photoreceptor region is rich in visible light, especially blue light. Primate and laboratory studies have shown that blue light, especially in the high-oxygen environment of the photoreceptors, causes damage to the RPE and choriocapillaris [6], resulting directly from the generation of ROS. Whether sunlight exposure in human populations is a risk factor for these conditions is more difficult to establish and relatively few studies have investigated this. Overall, the evidence suggests that high light exposures increase the risk of cataracts, especially cortical cataracts, with estimates of from 6 to 38% of cortical cataract being caused by sunlight exposure [7]. The evidence for AMD and light exposure is limited and inconclusive.

Genetic susceptibility

It is well established that a family history of AMD is a predisposition for this condition. However, only very recently have certain genes that confer a high risk of developing AMD been identified. To date the most consistent evidence is for genes that relate to the complement system, and a number of studies have now confirmed the association first reported two years ago [8]. Gene–environment interactions have also been shown, indicating synergistic effects, for example, between smoking and homozygosity [9]. Although twin and association studies [10] suggest that age-related cataract may also have a strong genetic component, no susceptibility genes have yet been identified.

Dietary factors

Antioxidants

The coincidence of onset of cataract and AMD in later life and age-related declines in antioxidant availability and activity led to the notion that deficiencies in antioxidants played a key role in the development of these conditions and, furthermore, that antioxidant supplementation might reduce their incidence or progression. *In vitro* and *in vivo* studies have demonstrated the important role of antioxidants in the lens and retina [6,11]. These include (1) the actions of the antioxidant enzymes, principally superoxide dismutase, catalase, glutathione, and glutathione peroxidase; and (2) the actions of the antioxidant vitamins: vitamins A, C, and E and the carotenoids, lutein and zeaxanthein. The antioxidant enzymes are the first-line defence system supported by the antioxidant vitamins. Vitamin C is the most important antioxidant vitamin in the lens and is found in the aqueous fluid at concentrations of thirty- to fifty-fold that of the plasma. In the macula, lutein and zeaxanthein are present in very high concentrations (as seen by the yellow spot). In addition to their antioxidant properties, lutein and zeaxanthein also filter blue light. Zinc is found in high concentrations in photoreceptors and RPE cells.

Difficulties in assessing the evidence in human populations are compounded by measurement errors (especially using dietary questionnaires), variations in reporting (e.g., by types of opacity [pure or mixed or any cataract]), information on nutritional levels and comparator groups (e.g., median, quartile, tertile), and subgroup analyses (mainly age and sex, and other risk factors). A number of reviews are available [11–13].

Some studies have found a protective association between vitamin C measured by diet intake and cataract [14,15], but other studies, including the large prospective Nurses Health Study, found no association [16,17]. Protective associations have been reported for vitamin C measured in plasma in case control studies in Mediterranean countries [18–20], but not in other case control studies [16,18,21]. One study found a protective effect of increased dietary intakes of vitamin E for cortical, nuclear, and mixed cataract [15], whilst there was again no association in the Nurses Health Study [17].

The evidence for a protective effect of vitamin E measured in the serum is stronger, with inverse associations reported for incident cataract in the Beaver Dam Eye Study [22] and with prevalent and incident nuclear cataract in the U.S.-based Lens Opacities Case Control Study [23,24]. Other studies have reported no association [18,19]. In the Nurses Health Study and the Health Professionals Study, weak negative associations with dietary carotenoids (mainly lutein and zeaxanthein) and cataract [25,26] were found. Further investigations of frequency of consumption of foods high in carotenoids—especially lutein (found in spinach and dark leafy green vegetables)—also showed protective associations with higher consumption [25,26]. Other studies have reported associations with serum levels of lutein and PSC [18] or no association of these carotenoids with any type of cataract [19,27].

No association has been found for dietary or plasma vitamin C with AMD [28–30]. Associations of serum alpha tocopherol or dietary vitamin E with AMD have been reported in some [28,31] but not all [30,32–34] studies. The Eye Disease Case Control Study found decreased risks of NVAMD with higher combined lutein/zeaxanthein concentrations [30]. A number of studies have examined associations between lutein and zeaxanthein and early ARM or with a combined end point of early ARM and NVAMD. The results from these studies are inconsistent.

Although the evidence does support a role for antioxidants in the aetiology of AMD and cataract, the evidence for one specific antioxidant over another is inconsistent and only partly accounted for by variations in study design and the methods used to assess antioxidant levels. It might be considered that variation in results between studies may reflect the different levels of antioxidants in the populations studied—for example, a stronger association in populations with low levels of a particular antioxidant. However, the strongest associations observed for vitamin C (based on plasma levels) and cataract were found in two studies from Mediterranean countries with high habitual levels of vitamin C [19,20]. Although there has been much promotion of lutein-rich foods, the evidence is equivocal [35].

The level of antioxidants required to protect the lens or retina is likely to depend on the level of exposures to external oxidative stress, such as light and smoking. Whilst most studies have adjusted for the confounding effects of these risk factors, there has been little attention to possible interactions between antioxidant levels and, for example, exposures to solar radiation and risk of cataract or AMD.

For the most part, studies have focused on one single antioxidant in exploring associations, although synergistic effects of antioxidants are well known. The few studies that have attempted to construct an overall antioxidant index or examined combinations of the key antioxidants have found inverse associations supporting the overall antioxidant hypothesis [36–38] For example, a high dietary intake of beta carotene, vitamins C and E, and zinc was associated with a substantially reduced risk of AMD in elderly persons in the Rotterdam Study [39].

Studies have also examined associations between patterns of diet. Fruit intake but not vegetable or carotenoid intake was inversely associated with the risk of NVAMD in the Health Professionals and Nurses Study [40]. A healthy eating index (HEI) was constructed based on adherence to recommended dietary guidelines for five food groups: grains, vegetables, fruit and fruit juice, milk and milk products, and meat (including fish, nuts, and dry beans). Women in the highest two quartiles of HEI had a 50% reduction in risk of lens opacities with no difference in effect between the third and top quartile; the effect was even stronger in nonusers of vitamin C supplements (around a 70% reduction in risk) [41]. However, it is difficult to be sure that adequate adjustment for confounding has been made in studies measuring healthy lifestyles. Similar concerns apply to studies showing supplement users were at decreased risk of cataract or AMD, thus prompting the need for evidence from unconfounded studies such as randomised controlled trials (RCTs).

The evidence from high-quality RCTs is limited, especially for AMD [42]. Only three trials to date have been specifically designed to evaluate the effects of supplementation on cataracts. No benefit was observed in the AREDS trial for high-dose antioxidant supplements (beta-carotene, vitamins C and E) on the development and progression of lens opacities [43]. The VECAT study found no reduction in incidence or progression of any type of cataract with high-dose vitamin E [44]. The only trial to demonstrate a benefit—the REACT study (beta carotene, vitamins C and E)—found a significant effect observed mainly in the U.S. centres. It is possible that the methods used to determine cataract progression in this trial had greater sensitivity than in the other trials [45]. For AMD, the strongest evidence of an effect of antioxidant supplementation is provided by the AREDS trial, which demonstrated that, amongst people with moderate signs of AMD at baseline, taking a high dose of multivitamins in combination with zinc was associated with an approximately 25% reduction in five-year progression [46].

Dietary fat

Dietary fat includes different subtypes such cholesterol and saturated and polyunsaturated fats, and there is substantial evidence from studies in diseases such as coronary heart disease that these fats have important adverse (e.g., saturated fats and cholesterol) or protective (e.g., polyunsaturated fats) health effects. In the eye disease case-control study there was some suggestion that high intakes of vegetable, monounsaturated, and polyunsaturated fats and linoleic acid (an n-6 PUFA) were associated with a greater risk for NVAMD [47], but the results were not clear-cut.

The photoreceptor membranes are rich in long chain polyunsaturated fatty acids, especially docosahexaenoic acid (DHA), the main source of which is marine oils. In laboratory studies, DHA has been shown to play an important role in a number of pathways that might plausibly influence the development of AMD [48], but the evidence from human studies is very limited [49]. A large RCT investigating the effect of supplementation with 1 g/day of omega-3 fatty acids or macular xanthophylls (lutein and zeaxanthein) supplements or both on progression of AMD or cataract is currently under way (http://www.nei.nih.gov/neitrials/viewStudyWeb.aspx?id=120).

Conclusions

Good vision is an essential component of independent living in later life. Cataract and age-related macular degeneration share a number of features common to age-related conditions: They occur rarely, if at all, before middle age and the prevalence rises with advancing age into the extremes of old age. Whilst AMD is not as prevalent as cataract, the effect on the individual is greater because of the lack of effective treatment for this condition. The strong and consistent association with smoking for both conditions as well as the multiplicative effects shown for genetically susceptible individuals for AMD highlights the importance of tobacco control policies and individual advice on smoking cessation.

Apart from people who already have moderately advanced AMD or AMD in one eye, supplement use is of no proven benefit for AMD. There is no evidence that supplements benefit cataracts. Until the results of further studies on omega-3 fatty acids are available, supplementation with these acids for the benefit of eye health is not indicated. The evidence does support, however, the consumption of an antioxidant-rich and varied diet that should also include oily fish as an important source of DHA. More definite recommendations for dietary means to tackle this important cause of age-associated disability and poor quality of life await the completion of several ongoing randomised controlled trials.

References

1. Congdon, N. et al., Causes and prevalence of visual impairment among adults in the United States. *Arch Ophthalmol*, 2004. 122(4):477–485.
2. Evans, J.R., A.E. Fletcher, and R.P. Wormald, Causes of visual impairment in people aged 75 years and older in Britain: An add-on study to the MRC Trial of Assessment and Management of Older People in the Community. *Br J Ophthalmol*, 2004. 88(3):365–370.
3. van Leeuwen, R. et al., The risk and natural course of age-related maculopathy: Follow-up at 6 1/2 years in the Rotterdam study. *Arch Ophthalmol*, 2003. 121(4):519–526.
4. Kelly, S.P. et al., Smoking and blindness. *BMJ*, 2004. 328(7439):537–538.
5. West, S., Does smoke get in your eyes? *JAMA*, 1992. 268(8):1025–1026.
6. Winkler, B.S. et al., Oxidative damage and age-related macular degeneration. *Mol Vis*, 1999. 5:32.
7. Oliva, M.S. and H. Taylor, Ultraviolet radiation and the eye. *Int Ophthalmol Clin*, 2005. 45(1):1–17.

8. Hageman, G.S. et al., A common haplotype in the complement regulatory gene factor H (HF1/CFH) predisposes individuals to age-related macular degeneration. *Proc Natl Acad Sci USA*, 2005. 102(20):7227–7232.
9. Despriet, D.D. et al., Complement factor H polymorphism, complement activators, and risk of age-related macular degeneration. *JAMA*, 2006. 296(3):301–309.
10. Hammond, C.J. et al., The heritability of age-related cortical cataract: The Twin Eye Study. *Invest Ophthalmol Vis Sci*, 2001. 42(3):601–605.
11. Taylor, A. and M. Hobbs, 2001 Assessment of nutritional influences on risk for cataract. *Nutrition*, 2001. 17(10):845–857.
12. Congdon, N.G. and K.P. West, Jr., Nutrition and the eye. *Curr Opin Ophthalmol*, 1999. 10(6):464–473.
13. Hogg, R. and U. Chakravarthy, AMD and micronutrient antioxidants. *Curr Eye Res*, 2004. 29(6):387–401.
14. Jacques, P.F. et al., Antioxidant status in persons with and without senile cataract. *Arch Ophthalmol*, 1988. 106(3):337–340.
15. Leske, M.C., L.T. Chylack, Jr., and S.Y. Wu, The Lens Opacities Case-Control Study. Risk factors for cataract. *Arch Ophthalmol*, 1991. 109(2):244–251.
16. Vitale, S. et al., Plasma antioxidants and risk of cortical and nuclear cataract. *Epidemiology*, 1993. 4(3):195–203.
17. Hankinson, S.E. et al., Nutrient intake and cataract extraction in women: A prospective study. *BMJ*, 1992. 305(6849):335–339.
18. Gale, C.R. et al., Plasma antioxidant vitamins and carotenoids and age-related cataract. *Ophthalmology*, 2001. 108(11):1992–1998.
19. Valero, M.P. et al., Vitamin C is associated with reduced risk of cataract in a Mediterranean population. *J Nutr*, 2002. 132(6):1299–1306.
20. Ferrigno, L. et al., Associations between plasma levels of vitamins and cataract in the Italian-American Clinical Trial of Nutritional Supplements and Age-Related Cataract (CTNS): CTNS report #2. *Ophthalmic Epidemiol*, 2005. 12(2):71–80.
21. Jacques, P.F. and L.T. Chylack, Jr., Epidemiologic evidence of a role for the antioxidant vitamins and carotenoids in cataract prevention. *Am J Clin Nutr*, 1991. 53(1 Suppl):352S–355S.
22. Lyle, B.J. et al., Serum carotenoids and tocopherols and incidence of age-related nuclear cataract. *Am J Clin Nutr*, 1999. 69(2):272–277.
23. Leske, M.C. et al., Biochemical factors in the lens opacities. Case-control study. The Lens Opacities Case-Control Study Group. *Arch Ophthalmol*, 1995. 113(9):1113–1119.
24. Leske, M.C. et al., Antioxidant vitamins and nuclear opacities: The longitudinal study of cataract. *Ophthalmology*, 1998. 105(5):831–836.
25. Brown, L. et al., A prospective study of carotenoid intake and risk of cataract extraction in U.S. men. *Am J Clin Nutr*, 1999. 70(4):517–524.
26. Chasan-Taber, L. et al., A prospective study of carotenoid and vitamin A intakes and risk of cataract extraction in U.S. women. *Am J Clin Nutr*, 1999. 70(4):509–516.
27. Delcourt, C. et al., Plasma lutein and zeaxanthin and other carotenoids as modifiable risk factors for age-related maculopathy and cataract: The POLA Study. *Invest Ophthalmol Vis Sci*, 2006. 47(6):2329–2335.

28. Delcourt, C. et al., Age-related macular degeneration and antioxidant status in the POLA study. POLA Study Group. Pathologies Oculaires Liees a l'Age. *Arch Ophthalmol*, 1999. 117(10):1384–1390.

29. West, S.V.S. et al., Are antioxidants or supplements protective for age-related macular degeneration? *Arch Ophthalmol*, 1994. 112:222–227.

30. The Eye Disease Case-Control Study Group, Antioxidant status and neovascular age-related macular degeneration. Eye Disease Case-Control Study Group. *Arch Ophthalmol*, 1993. 111(1):104–109.

31. West, S. et al., Are antioxidants or supplements protective for age-related macular degeneration? *Arch Ophthalmol*, 1994. 112(2):222–227.

32. Mares-Perlman, J.A. et al., Serum antioxidants and age-related macular degeneration in a population-based case-control study. *Arch Ophthalmol*, 1995. 113(12):1518–1523.

33. Smith, W., P. Mitchell, and C. Rochester, Serum beta carotene, alpha tocopherol, and age-related maculopathy: The Blue Mountains Eye Study. *Am J Ophthalmol*, 1997. 124(6):838–840.

34. Mares-Perlman, J.A. et al., Association of zinc and antioxidant nutrients with age-related maculopathy. *Arch Ophthalmol*, 1996. 114(8):991–997.

35. Mares-Perlman, J.A., Too soon for lutein supplements. *Am J Clin Nutr*, 1999. 70(4):431–432.

36. Delcourt, C. et al., Associations of cataract with antioxidant enzymes and other risk factors: The French Age-Related Eye Diseases (POLA) Prospective Study. *Ophthalmology*, 2003. 110(12):2318–2326.

37. Delcourt, C. et al., Associations of antioxidant enzymes with cataract and age-related macular degeneration. The POLA Study. Pathologies Oculaires Liees a l'Age. *Ophthalmology*, 1999. 106(2):215–222.

38. The Italian-American Cataract Study Group, Risk factors for age-related cortical, nuclear, and posterior subcapsular cataracts. *Am J Epidemiol*, 1991. 133(6):541–553.

39. van Leeuwen, R. et al., Dietary intake of antioxidants and risk of age-related macular degeneration. *JAMA*, 2005. 294(24):3101–3107.

40. Cho, E. et al., Prospective study of intake of fruits, vegetables, vitamins, and carotenoids and risk of age-related maculopathy. *Arch Ophthalmol*, 2004. 122(6):883–892.

41. Moeller, S.M. et al., Overall adherence to the dietary guidelines for Americans is associated with reduced prevalence of early age-related nuclear lens opacities in women. *J Nutr*, 2004. 134(7):1812–1819.

42. Evans, J.R., Antioxidant vitamin and mineral supplements for slowing the progression of age-related macular degeneration. *Cochrane Database Systematic Rev*, 2006(2):CD000254.

43. Age-Related Eye Disease Study, A randomized, placebo-controlled, clinical trial of high-dose supplementation with vitamins C and E and beta carotene for age-related cataract and vision loss: AREDS report no. 9. *Arch Ophthalmol*, 2001. 119(10):1439–1452.

44. McNeil, J.J. et al., Vitamin E supplementation and cataract: Randomized controlled trial. *Ophthalmology*, 2004. 111(1):75–84.

45. Chylack, L.T., Jr. et al., The Roche European American Cataract Trial (REACT): A randomized clinical trial to investigate the efficacy of an oral antioxidant micronutrient mixture to slow progression of age-related cataract. *Ophthalmic Epidemiol*, 2002. 9(1):49–80.

46. Age-Related Eye Disease Study Research Group, A randomized, placebo-controlled, clinical trial of high-dose supplementation with vitamins C and E, beta carotene, and zinc for age-related macular degeneration and vision loss: AREDS report no. 8. *Arch Ophthalmol*, 2001. 119:1417–1436.

47. Seddon, J.M. et al., Dietary fat and risk for advanced age-related macular degeneration. *Arch Ophthalmol*, 2001. 119(8):1191–1199.

48. SanGiovanni, J.P. and E.Y. Chew, The role of omega-3 long-chain polyunsaturated fatty acids in health and disease of the retina. *Prog Retin Eye Res*, 2005. 24(1):87–138.

49. Hodge, W. et al., Effects of omega-3 fatty acids on eye health. *Evid Rep Technol Assess* (Summ), 2005(117):1–6.

chapter five

Reminiscence in everyday talk between older people and their carers: implications for the quality of life of older people in care homes

Fiona Wilson, Kevin McKee, Helen Elford, Man Cheung Chung, Fiona Goudie, and Sharron Hinchliff

Contents

Introduction 36
Method...37
Results..38
    Level 1: Sharing lives and building relationships in
       everyday talk 38
    Level 2: Benefits of reminiscence in everyday talk...............................40
       Significance/feeling valued..40
       Intergenerational 41
    Level 3: Barriers and tensions..42
       Barriers and discontinuity 42
       Tensions in the caring role..44
       Tensions in using reminiscence 45
Discussion 46
    Main findings 46
       Maintaining self-identity through reminiscence.......................46
       Challenges in using reminiscence 47
       Supporting reminiscence in care homes 47

Conclusions and implications...48
Author note...49
References...49

Introduction

Writers and researchers frequently conceptualise reminiscence as a psycho-therapeutic process, citing Butler's [1] seminal work in which reminiscence is described in Eriksonian terms as a necessary and fundamental review of one's life in order to achieve fulfillment in old age [2]. In this tradition reminiscence is interpreted as an intrapersonal process that can occur spontaneously, but may be facilitated by those trained in reminiscence/counselling skills.

Formal reminiscence has also been presented as a useful tool with which to encourage social engagement, provide a sense of value to older people, and promote successful ageing. Woods and McKiernan [3] and Cheston [4], for example, describe reminiscence activities that encourage group discussion, expression, and communication, particularly for older people with some cognitive impairment. Thorsheim and Roberts [5] suggest that reminiscence can produce positive effects on health outcomes by increasing social support. Reminiscence in this tradition is seen as an interpersonal process. Reminiscence may therefore facilitate integrative (intrapersonal) and instrumental (interpersonal) processes [6]. This chapter aims to explore the functions of communication about the past and the present in everyday interactions between older people and their carers and evaluate the impact of past talk on their relationship and the quality of life of older people.

Exploration of the impact of reminiscence on caregiving relationships emphasises benefits to the delivery of formal caregiving. The use of life biography, for example [7–9], aims to facilitate individualised and person-centred approaches to caregiving in long-term care settings. Whilst Puentes [10] and Pulsford [11] are critical of reminiscence processes that appear to benefit staff in their role rather than directly supporting older people, there is support for reminiscence as an aid to fostering reciprocity in the caregiving relationship that is beneficial for carers and the older people they care for. Reciprocity refers to the well-established powerful normative obligation of a help recipient to assist people who have provided help to him or her [12,13]. Reciprocity as discussed by Nolan and Keady [9] is an approach to caregiving that stresses the importance of past, present, and future in caring relationships. Lewinter (cited in Nolan et al. [14]), in an empirical study of reciprocity between older people and home helps in Denmark, found that home helps were rewarded by feeling needed and appreciated by their clients and in turn found time to listen to and value the contributions of the older person.

Other studies discuss the direct benefits of informal reminiscence for older people, with emphasis on narrative and discourse as a means for forging social relationships and preserving self-identity. This is seen as particularly important in the transition to a formal care setting. For example, Froggatt [15], in work on self-identify in residential settings in England, concludes that there is 'sequestration' of individuals—a social death on entering care settings. However, Reed and Payton [16] challenge this negative portrayal of older people in care settings, arguing that older people actively 'construct familiarity', forging strong relationships with each other and staff through everyday talk. Here, reminiscence is described as a social, everyday activity in which residents rediscovered and made acquaintances through familiar reference points such as neighbourhood, work history, and so forth. Again, Newton [17] notes the role of past talk for residents in a residential home in maintaining continuity with the outside world and with other residents and staff. In this sense, reminiscence facilitates and forms part of a process of 'coauthoring' by the negotiation of self and identity in a care environment [18].

Reminiscence assumes a focus on the past. However, discursive approaches that focus on identity and relationships suggest that the past requires some continuum with the present. In a study on the interaction between the self and the meaning of objects and environments, Rubenstein [19] concludes that 'in a sense reminiscence was a form of attachment, not to the past but to persons and places still germane in the present' (p. 155). For Randall and Kenyon [18], the narrative environment is important in shaping identity and self and therefore 'the machinery of everyday conversation…provides the scaffolding that supports the discursive practice which constitutes selves' (p. 238).

This chapter reports results from a study designed to evaluate whether engaging in reminiscence has an impact on the quality of life of frail older people. As part of this study, over a period of twelve months, a series of focus groups were conducted with older people resident in eighteen care settings in Sheffield, United Kingdom, and their formal and informal carers. The key aim of this qualitative component of the study was to explore the role of reminiscence in everyday interactions between older people in care settings and their carers.

Method

Using a complete list of residential and nursing homes and older people day-care centres within Sheffield city boundaries, thirty-four potential fieldwork sites were initially selected via a sampling frame designed to ensure representation of all areas of the city and all major care providers. Of these sites, eighteen were recruited.

Seven focus groups were conducted in total, in which care staff, residents, and residents' relatives from all eighteen fieldwork sites were represented. Two care staff groups (comprising four and six staff members) were conducted with staff from residential and nursing homes. One group consisted of seven activity workers from a mix of care settings, one group

($n = 14$) with older residents, and one informal carers' group ($n = 5$). Two mixed groups of older residents and care staff (with thirteen and twelve participants, the first comprising seven older people and six care staff, the second comprising eight older people and four care staff) were also conducted.

A moderator and one observer facilitated focus group sessions. All sessions were audio taped and observations recorded, and they lasted on average approximately one hour. An interview schedule was developed, and four main topic areas were used as prompts for discussion: when do you talk about the present and past or future; who to; where; and what are the benefits or drawbacks to talking about the present and the past?

The audiotapes of the focus groups were transcribed in full and subjected to interpretative phenomenological analysis [20]. This approach differs from that of discourse analysis in that the researcher is not concerned with the talk or discourse but the underlying cognition—what the participant thinks or believes about the topic under discussion. Analysis of data was assisted by Nudist 6 and emergent themes explored by the research team. A table of master themes was used to map and elucidate the dynamics and relationships between themes.

Results

Emergent themes related to three interlinked levels (Figure 5.1). The first level focuses on everyday interactions (including talk about past and present) in order to build relationships, whilst the second level explores the function of interactions entirely grounded in talk about the past. The third level explores the barriers and underlying tensions in talking about the past and present in everyday interactions including barriers to identity management and organisational constraints. Each level and the associated themes will be discussed in turn.

Level 1: Sharing lives and building relationships in everyday talk

At the first level, one key function of the past and present in everyday talk was the building of relationships and the sharing of lives, and this establishing of reciprocity was important in identity maintenance and negotiation of self (Figure 5.2).

Sharing lives demands a strong sense of self-identity in order to enable reciprocity amongst older people, their families, and their carers; this was essential in maintaining a sense of continuity of self, community, and family and in keeping in touch with the world generally. Reciprocity provided older people and carers with a sense of continuity and generativity between past and present. Transgenerational talk focused on universal themes, such as the family, and enabled staff and older people to talk about their lives in mutually supportive ways:

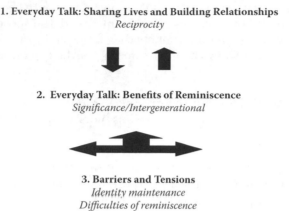

1. Everyday Talk: Sharing Lives and Building Relationships
Reciprocity

2. Everyday Talk: Benefits of Reminiscence
Significance/Intergenerational

3. Barriers and Tensions
Identity maintenance
Difficulties of reminiscence
Organizational constraints

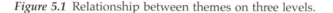

Figure 5.1 Relationship between themes on three levels.

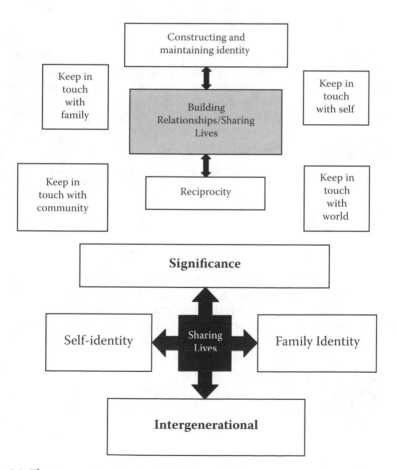

Figure 5.2 Themes on two levels: detailed analysis.

> Yes, you can talk to them about their own experience about what's happening to you, and they're really interested. I suppose it works both ways, knowing that somebody's interested in what's going off in our life; it shows they care, doesn't it? (Jane,* care staff focus group)

The sharing of lives and self operated around talk in the past and the present and was used by carers as well as older people. One male member of staff commented:

> Reflecting on the past, learning about the things that were there when we weren't, and sharing those memories. In fact, I sometimes share my own memories. It sometimes helps to bring down barriers doesn't it, if there's a barrier between you and a resident? (John, care staff, mixed focus group of care staff and residents)

Building relationships indicates a search for common ground, and this was particularly so between older people and their peers:

> We have two residents who had the same job—they were both firemen so when the other one came in he actually knew this man. It was unbelievable and so we took them in and it was great. They got on like a house on fire. It was lovely. After that they got really friendly and both had someone to talk to…as soon as we said this gentleman was coming and that he knew them, he came out of himself, unbelievable. (Maria, care staff focus group)

This illustrates how past and present are inextricably linked and how the past can be used as a reference point to form familiarity or common ground in the present.

Level 2: Benefits of reminiscence in everyday talk

Informal talk that focussed entirely on the past could bestow a strong sense of significance and feeling of value. Intergenerationality, the role of reminiscence across generations, also indicated that reminiscence can provide a sense of identity and significance to older people and their families (Figure 5.2).

Significance/feeling valued

One activity worker illustrated how acknowledging the past helps care staff to recognise the significance of past lives and promote self-esteem in the older person:

---

* Participants' names following quotations have been changed to preserve anonymity.

> Taking the lady over there...she actually takes pride in the fact that she did her little bit, she was in the war, er, so little things like that, yes, you do boost the self esteem, because she's telling me that at a certain period in time, she played a key role. (John, care staff, mixed focus group of care staff and residents)

The resident in question commented that listening and attentiveness are key in this process of giving significance:

> But if I am speaking to someone who seems really impressed—What an ambulance? With all the bombs coming down? But it all depends on whether the person you're speaking to is bothered or not. (Edna, resident, mixed focus group of care staff and residents)

Through attentiveness and listening, the uniqueness of an individual could be heard and understood, indicating a continuum of self between past to present. One activity worker noted:

> Through the past you get to see more of them as a person because they're not a condition that's come in for you to look after, they are people, and the more you get to know them, the more you relate to them don't you? And it helps you to understand why they might do things that they do now because of what's happened in the past, or how they may have reacted to things in the past. (Mary, activity worker focus group)

Intergenerational

Links with the past enabled older people to give a sense of significance and identity to carers, including paid staff and family. Family folklore or genealogy particularly fascinated family carers. In many ways, the older person acted as the keeper of family folklore and this history gave a unique sense of significance and identity to all family members:

> Well, even when you are little with your own parents, you like to hear stories of when your mum and dad were little, and they would become part of your family folklore. Only now everyone doesn't now sit round the fire and talk—they're all off doing computer games or whatever. There is a danger of those stories being lost in a way. But at the end of the day, it's just fascinating really, like when you like to look at old photographs. (Mary, activity worker focus group)

The past also reached across generations, too, as illustrated by this response to a written biography completed by one older resident as part of guided reminiscence activity:

...when her grandkids come in and they're doing Victorian times, and they sat there reading through her book—'did they really have that when you were little?' This little girl is about seven and she can't imagine her grandmother being seven. You can see it ticking over in her head. But they're really beginning to connect, you know. (Sylvia, activity worker focus group)

Older people can therefore provide transgenerational benefits by offering identity and cultural values to those around them. Certainly, those carers and older people involved in the study valued the sharing of everyday talk around transgenerational issues, particularly family and children. Older people in the study gained significance as the 'keepers' of family folklore knowledge and history.

Level 3: Barriers and tensions

Whilst everyday interaction involving past and present talk was essential in maintaining a sense of self and in facilitating caregiving relationships, there were barriers and tensions present in the discussions (Figure 5.1). Carers and older people recognised a number of challenges and these included the ability or inability to negotiate identity and build relationships, as well as organisational factors that impinge on the caregiving role. These manifest as a sense of discontinuity experienced by older people and in tensions in the care role.

Barriers and discontinuity

Discontinuity of self focussed on issues around loss of identity that might be precipitated by barriers such as disability, loss of peers, or a move into a home. Hearing impairment or loss of memory, for example, can inhibit social and interpersonal interaction:

I think mother is aware that she's actually losing it a bit, and I think she feels embarrassed getting into a conversation with people she doesn't know, because (a) as you say she doesn't know this area, but (b) she realises that she's getting a bit confused. But she's been sitting at a table with three other ladies since September and she still can't remember their names. (son of resident, relatives' focus group)

There was a sense of discontinuity as comrades and friends diminished. Carers or younger family seemed unable to 'connect' and provide the comradeship and familiarity of the past. Some family carers appeared to recognise this, seeking out peer groups for their older relative:

I did used to take him down to talk with his friends; they were all miners, they'd all worked at the same pit, and they used to talk for hours. I'd sit him with his mates he'd worked with all his life, and they'd sit and they'd chat and that was all right, but in the latter stages when I took him down, there he didn't know anybody; he'd say, 'Who's that'? And the problems were that I didn't know who they were either, you see? (daughter of resident, relatives' focus group)

Feelings of dislocation and being cut off from the world that derived from living in a care home setting also gave rise to a sense of discontinuity:

There's many a time—well, most nights—I'll sit out on the front for ten minutes and thought about running away. I felt I was in a remand home. I hate feeling locked in, and I don't know, I suppose there are other people in the same boat...but it is me that's locked in. (Sam, resident, mixed focus group of care staff and residents)

Comfort zone.   Care staff recognised that feelings of dislocation may precipitate a return to the past as a comfort zone:

I do I think they love it [reminiscence]. They don't get out that often, so they're cut off from the world kind of thing, but their world that they remember is the past, so therefore that's what they enjoy. (Joan, care staff focus group)

Whilst a comfort zone may offer a safe haven, in many ways it represents a further aspect of discontinuity expressed as a rift between past and present. There was a sense in which, for older people, the present was not *their* world, but hostile and lonely. A hostile present precipitated a return to the past:

If he said for some reason or another he wanted to go home, he wasn't talking about where we were living, he wasn't talking about where I'd moved him from where they'd lived for sixty years, he was talking about his childhood as a little boy. He wanted to go back to where he was a little boy. (daughter of resident, relatives' focus group)

This was reflected in the continual comparison between past and present, in which the past was always presented more favourably than the present:

I wouldn't like to relive my life again, not in this world. The world's all right but it's the people that live in it—villains and vicious people. They'll do anything for money now—murder, tie pensioners up. (Fred, resident, older persons' focus group)

Tensions in the caring role

Tensions within the caring role impinged upon the role of everyday talk as a therapeutic medium with which to counter discontinuity. A key barrier to everyday talk and reminiscence was organisational constraints that produced tensions in the caregiving role. Chatting was implicitly recognised as an important aspect of social care, but organisational constraints emphasised physical over social care. Both care staff and older people identified time constraints as obstacles to social interaction:

> I think it's more frustrating if you want to spend that time with them, and listen to them, and you know you haven't got time to. I think that's what's frustrating about it, because even though they might have told you yesterday, obviously the something that's that important to them, they just want you to listen. (Jean, care staff focus group)

Some staff managed the tensions between social and physical care by incorporating both together:

> You know if somebody has been really down…I have actually said this person could really do with a bath, just to spend time with them you know. I've actually done that, I really have. And then probably spent longer than I should have in the bathroom with them, you know just to spend that bit of time with them. (Jane, care staff focus group)

The overlapping of the physical with the social was recognised by older people too:

> Researcher: When do you talk to care staff?

> Resident: Well, when you are having a bath normally because they are so busy, they can't be listening to you all the time can they? (Elsie, older persons' focus group)

Achieving a balance of physical and social care required privacy and intimacy, and meaningful everyday interactions with residents were more prevalent when care staff members were engaged in intimate caring tasks. Social care in this context represented quality time.

Overload.   The sharing of lives, whilst commendable in supporting person-centred care approaches, did blur boundaries. There were examples of care staff and older people meeting on staff days off or care staff introducing their families, inviting older residents home for dinner, and often buying clothes and presents. Whilst going the extra mile might seem laudable, some staff expressed a feeling of overload, resentment, and lack of support. One care worker with two small children recounted:

> I can be working six days one week with five weeks and one day off. And this particular resident wanted to go for lunch…'for three weeks I've been asking', you know. So I thought, I'll actually do it, and so it meant I'd worked seven days, and I was absolutely shattered…. (Sophie, care staff focus group)

Tensions in using reminiscence

Activity workers tended to avoid obvious reminiscence activities but opted instead for group activities that might allow reminiscence. Interestingly, few offered one-to-one activities; rather, one-to-one interactions tended to occur as care staff went about their duties. The difficulties identified by staff in group reminiscence are similar to those encountered in group work generally and included intolerance of other group members (particularly those with confusion) and personality conflicts. Reminiscence was rarely used in activity sessions as a key topic but activity workers talked of reminiscence being 'wheedled' in. There was an implicit belief that older people would perceive formal reminiscence activities as patronizing:

> I must admit I wouldn't call a session reminiscence, but all sessions, reminiscence is involved in it. You are constantly reminiscing through the session, but I don't know whether it would put them off. (Cathy, activity worker focus group)

Recognising that formal or contrived reminiscence was difficult, care staff also recognised that spontaneous interactions around the past could be unpredictable, and there was fear that the past may evoke distressing memories and 'open wounds':

> Some things in the past upset people so we try not to mention them, but sometimes it's good because if they couldn't talk about it, they've kept something hidden inside for perhaps thirty or forty years, and then you've just opened it up again haven't you? So I suppose you have to be careful because once you've triggered something off—I mean you just go home don't you at the end of the day? (Mary, care staff focus group)

In many ways, talk about general everyday topics avoided evaluative or distressing dialogue about the past. Talk about children and families was preferred as a much safer topic by older people and care staff. Whilst such talk may help to build relationships, there is a danger that everyday talk using platitude may make meaningful interactions impossible. This was evident, for example, in residents' experience of dislocation and in the notion of a comfort zone. In one focus group, a resident expressed loss and the feeling of being trapped, which the care staff attempted to override and gloss over.

Present talk.   One of the key questions in the focus groups was around talk to do with the present and older people and carers positively advocated this. Many older residents enjoyed new challenges and activities. Valued examples cited included exercise classes, general social events involving family, and new challenges such as karaoke, jogging, day trips, line dancing, and computers; with glee, one focus group discussed some strippers who had visited the residential home. One activity worker concentrated on one-to-one work, keying into individual hobbies and facilitating interests such as managing shares on the stock market, art, and travel abroad to family. This raises the question of whether a strong focus on reminiscence and the past undermines the expression of self in the present and actually creates discontinuity rather than continuity. Nevertheless, the past may offer a key to continuity; for example, one carer identified swimming as a past passion for an older disabled person and organised swimming sessions with positive results. Everyday talk including a past and a present focus was important in maintaining a sense of self-identity and for keeping in touch with community and family.

Discussion

Main findings

In general, everyday interaction provides opportunities for carers and older people to open up channels of communication; enable relationships; and promote significance, self-esteem, and psychological health for older people. Interaction or activities that build on the past but are situated in the present offer opportunities for positive interaction, and past and present talk offer ways of overcoming discontinuity. However, a focus on just the past or just the present undermines self-identity and continuity of self, for we are all of the past and the present.

Maintaining self-identity through reminiscence

Giddens [21] discusses self-identify in existentialist terms linking biography, integrity, and continuity and argues that the person who is able to maintain a self-identify 'has a feeling of biographical continuity which she is able to grasp reflexively and, to a greater or lesser degree, communicate to other people' (p. 54). Everyday talk is therefore important in maintaining and developing a sense of self and can be described as a therapeutic medium for the cared for and the carer. Therapeutic talk is not confined to past talk and Coleman et al. [22] emphasise the importance of past, present, and future, arguing that a theme around self-identity 'may be constituted from elements of both past and present' (p. 158).

Reminiscence in everyday talk also demonstrated the potential for identity maintenance because the need to express who we are and relate to others can constitute a reciprocal relationship with peers and between older people and carers. Reminiscence also permits transgenerational benefits that offer significance to older people and their carers. Coleman et al. [22], for example, argue that 'it is clear that reminiscence serves social needs as well. It produces optimum effects where it has social benefits as well [as psychological benefits], particularly through the transmission of cultural values' (p. 221). Certainly, carers and older people involved in the study valued the sharing of everyday talk around transgenerational issues, particularly family and children.

Challenges in using reminiscence

The concept of reminiscence as a clearly defined therapy with a skilled professional dedicated to that aim was not apparent in the homes visited. Care staff and family carers did, however, demonstrate excellent intuitive skills. Within that intuition was an implicit recognition of discontinuities between past self and present self, tensions within the caring role, and recognition of the barriers and benefits to reminiscence (particularly in caring for older people with cognitive impairment). Whilst carers and older people identified the importance of everyday talk, there was a danger that potentially difficult conversations might be avoided. There was little mention, for example, of death or loss or fear; whilst the focus groups may not have been conducive to expression on such topics, there was a danger that avoidance of difficult topics might result in platitude and lack of opportunity for people to discuss meaningful emotions in the present. Avoidance of difficult interactions may result in an emphasis on the past as a comfort zone and this supports Coleman's writing [23] on disengagement in which people return to the familiar 'as a means of maintaining a coherent sense of one's self in later life, particularly in stressful situations such as relocation' (p. 86).

Platitudes also emanated from older people, perhaps suggesting that a reciprocal relationship with a paid worker was not always desirable. Whilst the dynamics within joint focus groups of older people and care staff indicated a sense of solidarity, there was evidence from carers that occasionally comradeship between older people was based on a familiarity or past reference point with which it was difficult for carers to engage. Moreover, an emphasis on the past in everyday talk assumes an offered biography to support a relationship between older person and carer, and yet many may not wish to trade their biography to facilitate a caring relationship. Perhaps this might explain why activity sessions that focused explicitly on reminiscence were avoided.

Supporting reminiscence in care homes

Enabling staff to use reminiscence as a way of developing reciprocal interactions with the older people they care for may be a useful way of improving the quality of life of older people in residential settings. However, the capacity of family carers or care staff to act as therapists at a formal or an informal level is questionable. Staden [24] argues that care work denotes emotional labour that is difficult to articulate and many workers are unable to list the skills employed in such work, maintaining a belief that the capacity to engage in emotional labour is simply absorbed through life experience. Bornat et al. [25] evaluated a pilot study of reminiscence in care settings and similarly concluded that staff members were generally unsupported and did not have access to training with which to facilitate interactions around reminiscence at formal or informal levels.

Everyday interactions were described as spontaneous opportunities for supportive interaction. However, there was recognition of organisational constraints, particularly regarding time, and an emphasis on bathing as an almost clandestine means of obtaining 'quality time' in the formal care setting. Twigg's work [26] similarly notes that humanist approaches are constrained by managerialist moves towards 'cost effectiveness' and her work on the 'social bath' suggests that, indeed, physical work is often regarded as legitimate whilst social care is disregarded as wasting time. In addition, carers and older people expressed unease regarding role boundaries (issues of confidentiality and staff working on days off) and organisational support in dealing with difficult interactions.

Conclusions and implications

It would seem that everyday talk encompassing past, present, and future provides an opportunity for a reciprocal, relationship-centred focus on caregiving that offers benefits in terms of social interaction, identity, and well-being to family carers, care staff, and older people. Present and past talk is inextricable and both may be therapeutic but also confrontational. Facilitating staff to harness everyday interactions requires support and training as well as managerial recognition of the importance of social care and 'chatting'. Similar recommendations have been broadly made [9,25,27].

This organisational framework should recognise the importance of social interaction as well as the individuality and needs of those involved. A positive emphasis on social care, making explicit the skills involved in 'just talking', must also ensure that the sole focus of talk is not reminiscence alone. Indeed, a focus on the past in some way precludes older people from addressing discontinuities that may be present in their lives here and now. Reed and Payton [26] write that, regarding the construction of familiarity by older people, 'rather than dwelling on the discontinuities that life in the care home might represent to them; failing health, loss of confidence and inability to manage daily chores, they appear to work at building bridges between their past and present life experiences' (p. 559). A consideration of discontinuity and the sorts of issues and skills involved in talking meaningfully about the past and present may facilitate more beneficial interactions, supporting the process of ageing well for older people and improving their quality of life, together with their carers, in home and formal care settings.

Author note

The research reported in this chapter was funded by a grant from the Economic and Social Research Council (Award No.: L480254031) as part of the Growing Older programme. The research was carried out in accordance with the BPS ethical guidelines for research and received approval from the North Sheffield Research Ethics Committee.

References

1. Butler, R.N. The life review: An interpretation of reminiscence in the aged. *Psychiatry,* 256, 65, 1963.
2. Woods, B. et al. Reminiscence and life review with persons with dementia: Which way forward? In: *Care-Giving in Dementia*, vol. 1, ed. Miesen, B.M.L and Jones, G.M.M. Routledge, London, 1992, 137.
3. Woods, B. and McKiernan, F. Evaluating the impact of reminiscence on older people with dementia. In: *The Art and Science of Reminiscing: Theory, Research, Methods and Applications*, ed. Haight, B.K. and Webster, J.D. Taylor & Francis, Philadelphia, 1995, 233.
4. Cheston, R. Psychotherapeutic work with people with dementia: A review of the literature. *Br J Med Psychol*, 71, 211, 1998.
5. Thorsheim, H.I. and Roberts, B. Finding common ground and mutual social support through reminiscing and telling one's story. In: *The Art and Science of Reminiscing: Theory, Research, Methods and Applications*, ed. Haight, B.K. and Webster, J.D. Taylor & Francis, Philadelphia, 1995, 193.
6. Wong, P.T.P. and Watt, L.M. What types of reminiscence are associated with successful aging? *Psychol Aging*, 6, 272, 1991.
7. Adams, J., Bornat, J., and Prickett, M. 'You wouldn't be interested in my life, I've done nothing'. Care planning and life-history work with frail older women. In: *Reviewing Care Management for Older People*, ed. Phillips, J. and Penhale, B. Jessica Kingsley Publishers, London, 1996, 102.
8. Chamberlayne, P. and King, A. The biographical challenge of caring. *Sociol Health Ill*, 19, 601, 1997.
9. Nolan, M. and Keady, J. Training in long-term care: The road to better quality. *Rev Clin Gerontol*, 6, 333, 1996.
10. Puentes, W.J. Using social reminiscence to teach therapeutic communication skills. *Geriatr Nurs*, 21, 315, 2000.
11. Pulsford, D. Therapeutic activities for people with dementia—What, why…and why not? *J Adv Nurs*, 26, 704, 1997.
12. Gouldner, A.W. The norm of reciprocity: A preliminary statement. *Am Sociol Rev*, 25, 161, 1960.
13. Antonucci, T.C. Social support and social relationships. In: *Handbook of Aging and the Social Sciences*, 3rd ed., ed. Binstock, R. and George, L. Academic Press, San Diego, CA, 1990, 205.

14. Nolan, M., Davies, S., and Grant, G. Quality of life, quality of care. In: *Working with Older People and Their Families,* ed. Nolan, M., Davies, S., and Grant, G. Open University Press, Buckingham, 2001, 4.

15. Froggatt, K. Life and death in English nursing homes: Sequestration or transition? *Ageing Soc,* 21, 319, 2001.

16. Reed, J. and Payton, V.R. Constructing familiarity and managing the self: Ways of adapting to life in nursing and residential homes for older people. *Ageing Soc,* 16, 543, 1996.

17. Newton, J. The geographical experience of older people in a residential home in South Yorkshire. *Generations Rev,* 9(2), 8, 1999.

18. Randall, L.W. and Kenyon, M.G. Reminiscence as reading our lives: Towards a wisdom environment. In: *Critical Advances in Reminiscence Work: From Theory to Application,* ed. Webster, J.D. and Haight, B.K. Springer Publishing Company, New York, 2002, 233.

19. Rubenstein, L.R. Reminiscence, personal meaning, themes and the 'object relations' of older people. In: *Critical Advances in Reminiscence Work: From Theory to Application,* ed. Webster, J.D. and Haight, B.K. Springer Publishing Company, New York, 2002, 153.

20. Smith, J.A. Beyond the divide between cognition and discourse. Using interpretative phenomenological analysis in health psychology. *Psychol Health,* 11, 261, 1996.

21. Giddens, A. *Modernity and Self-identity: Self and Society in the Late Modern Age,* Polity Press, Cambridge, 1991.

22. Coleman, P.G., Hautamaki, A., and Podloskij, A. Trauma, reconciliation, and generativity: The stories told by European war veterans. In: *Critical Advances in Reminiscence Work: From Theory to Application,* ed. Webster, J.D. and Haight, B.K. Springer Publishing Company, New York, 2002, 218.

23. Coleman, P. Psychological ageing. In: *Ageing in Society: An Introduction to Social Gerontology,* 2nd ed., ed. Bond, J., Coleman, P., and Peace, S. Sage Publications, London, 1993, 68.

24. Staden, H. Alertness to the needs of others: A study of the emotional labour of caring. *J Adv Nurs,* 27, 147, 1998.

25. Bornat, J. *Redefining Reminiscence in Care Settings.* Centre for Biography in Social Policy (BISP), University of East London, 1998.

26. Twigg, J. Carework as a form of bodywork. *Ageing Soc,* 20, 389, 2000.

27. Henwood, M. *Future Imperfect? Report of the King's Fund Care and Support Inquiry.* King's Fund Publishing, London, 2001.

chapter six

Retention of cognitive function in old age: why initial intelligence is important

Lawrence J. Whalley

Contents

Summary 51
Introduction 52
    Three key principles in ageing research 53
    The value of childhood (or initial) intelligence (IQ)...........................53
    Cognitive reserve and a threshold for dementia..............................53
    Adaptive and compensatory responses to brain ageing.....................54
    The role of personality 55
The Scottish Mental Surveys..56
    Major risk factors 57
    Molecular genetic studies..58
    Nutritional studies..59
    Health-related behaviours 61
Conclusions..63
References...63

Summary

The role of initial intelligence in the retention of cognitive function is important for two reasons. First, measures of initial intelligence provide a baseline from which the rate of change in function with age can be estimated. When this baseline is known, it makes more feasible the detection of factors (genetic or environmental) that may influence rates of cognitive change. These factors may be protective (as is claimed for education) or hazardous (as for hypertension). Knowing initial intelligence helps avoid presuming that an influence associated with variation in level of cognitive performance with age is attributable to ageing when there may be good reason to relate variation in level in later life with variation in initial intelligence (baseline). Second, intelligence influences the development of certain useful cognitive styles associated with the acquisition of strategies that promote retention of cognitive performance. This chapter reviews some aspects of the contributions made through follow-up studies of the Scottish Mental Surveys of 1932 and 1947. Molecular genetic, nutritional, and health-related behaviours are selected for inclusion in this chapter because they reflect the application of key principles in ageing research to understanding major determinants of ageing well and, potentially, a better understanding of sources of health inequalities in old age.

Introduction

In addition to the absence of age-related physical disabilities, ageing well requires retention of general mental ability to support continuing quality of life. This chapter first examines some of the conceptual foundations underpinning the scientific study of the role of intelligence in retention of cognitive ability. Second, the proposed conceptual framework supports an analysis of how and why individual differences in cognitive processes arise in late adulthood and old age. Third, our studies on the influence of childhood intelligence on many aspects of ageing are reviewed. The aim of these studies is to explore the nature of and extent to which important underlying influences account for differences in rates of cognitive ageing. The studies show how childhood intelligence can be used as a baseline from which to estimate lifelong cognitive change, and this is illustrated using our findings from molecular genetic studies. Choices about dietary habits and food supplement use are made in the light of cultural practices, relative costs, energy requirements, knowledge about nutrient values, and personal preferences. Trait intelligence, to which childhood intelligence contributes about 50%, informs many of these choices.

In the second illustration from our work, observational studies on the association in old people between blood micronutrients and cognitive functions are summarised. The impact of food supplement use on cognition is also presented. In the final illustration, childhood intelligence is considered as a novel risk factor for a number of age-related disorders, including coronary heart disease, cerebrovascular disease, and stroke. Although childhood intelligence can explain part of the well-established association between low social class and increased morbidity and mortality, it does not provide a complete explanation. Other factors must be at work.

Three key principles in ageing research

The National Institute of Ageing Working Group on Ageing and Genetic Epidemiology argued for the adoption of three principles in ageing research [1]. First, it is necessary to identify and then distinguish between those factors that determine survival up to becoming an old person. Failure to do this may confound important determinants of survivorship with influences on ageing itself [2,3]. Second, it is valuable to distinguish between an optimum or 'baseline' level of performance achieved in physiological or cognitive function across the life course and, later, rate of change over a specified age interval within old age. Third, once rates of change in selected parameters have been established, after adjustment for baseline, it is informative to relate such rates of change to changes in pathological parameters linked to possible fundamental sources of individual differences in rates of ageing.

In this chapter, these principles are explored in the context of cognitive ageing. Here, initial or 'premorbid' intelligence measures, obtained in childhood, provide a useful baseline against which rates of change in general or specific cognitive abilities can be measured over specified age intervals. In the final section of this chapter, a novel influence of childhood intelligence on age-related diseases is introduced. The possibility is raised that intelligence may affect the pathogenesis of age-related disease through its relationships with the efficiency of central regulatory systems that serve to maintain bodily integrity in the face of external perturbations.

The value of childhood (or initial) intelligence (IQ)

Knowing childhood IQ is useful in cognitive ageing research because it provides a baseline against which any later cognitive variation may be estimated [4]. Such data are rarely available in large population-based samples and, when IQ data are available, they most often include only men whose IQs were measured on induction to military service. Some models of cognitive variation with ageing seek proxies for the capacity of the brain to withstand insult or injury, including the neuropathologies of ageing. Researchers studying mental development in later life are often able to collect data at different time points. These repeated observations allow estimation of age-related change within old age. Sometimes, repeated observations do not interfere with the phenomena under inspection (e.g., of a physical measure such as girth) but in the case of mental abilities, repeated testing can produce improvements related to practice or to a disinclination to be retested and failure to remain in the study. Initial (or childhood) intelligence is one of several positive influences on improvement with practice.

Cognitive reserve and a threshold for dementia

At some point between ages of about eighteen and thirty years in early adulthood, maximum or optimal performance is attained in most cognitive abilities. Thereafter, there is a shallow decline in most abilities from about thirty to forty years of age and this gathers pace from age about sixty years and thereafter on into late old age. A subgroup of individuals will encounter catastrophic rates of cognitive decline, passing through a threshold of cognitive function, below which the capacity for independent life is jeopardised. This is sometimes termed the 'dementia threshold'. Such a schema also suggests that individuals vary in the extent to which they must decline in order to cross such a threshold. This variation, used to buffer the impact on the ageing brain of disease and neurodegenerative processes, is termed the 'cognitive reserve' [5], but as shown later, this should not be understood as the equivalent of childhood intelligence.

There are positive and negative genetic and environmental influences on the attainment of maximum cognitive threshold. The following discussion of the influences of childhood intelligence on the retention of cognitive function will focus on the role of intelligence in the acquisition of health-related behaviours, the use of health services, and the importance of retention of social and intellectual engagement as determining influences on the retention of cognitive ability. Put succinctly, intelligence may reflect intrinsic cognitive reserve and may also, over the life course, shape the external environment [6].

Adaptive and compensatory responses to brain ageing

The ageing brain is subject to three important harmful influences that determine some of the individual variation in cognitive ageing [7]. First, intrinsic and extrinsic antioxidant defences become less efficient in protecting brain cells from the impact of oxidative stress. Ageing brain cell function is compromised by processes connected with a low-grade brain inflammatory response. These processes accompany local metabolic changes that trigger 'programmed cell death' (apoptosis) in susceptible brain cells. The brain and mental processes do not respond passively to this loss of brain processing power and there are many interacting levels of adaptive and compensatory response available to the ageing brain. The recruitment of neural networks to undertake brainwork previously done by now damaged, ageing brain cells is one measurable component of the brain's compensatory response. Such cortical reorganisation may be underpinned by reinstatement of molecular mechanisms that determine embryonic and later neurogenesis [8].

Cognitive processes may contribute in subtle but significant ways to adaptive and/or compensatory responses. It is attractive to envisage the ageing mind applying existing cognitive structures and processes to the problems posed by the ageing brain. In support of this, much evidence points to the importance of an engaged, adaptive social lifestyle in the maintenance of cognitive functions in late life [9]. Likewise, lifelong occupational complexity appears to be important in developing the mental capacity to withstand the effects of ageing on the brain. Original or initial intelligence is a major influence on choice of recreational pursuits. Higher average intelligence is associated with the choice of recreations that are mentally effortful, perhaps indicating the continuity of the lifelong effects of intelligence on educational attainments, job choice, and the taking up of opportunities for later education and occupational retraining.

The role of personality

The assumption is not yet well-founded that childhood intelligence is a dominant influence on rates of cognitive ageing, and many other major factors exist. For example, some personality traits may place constraints on the opportunities for social engagement; low agreeableness or extremes of conscientiousness may reduce an individual's 'attractiveness' and impair an individual's capacity to sustain long-term social relationships leading to impoverishment of the social supports available to counter stressors or age-related cognitive decline [10].

Personality traits are internal mental processes with the capacity to influence acquisition of many adaptive behaviours in late life. In addition to sustained intellectual and social engagement, an individual's efficiency in responding to physical change (sensory loss, decreased mobility, the impact of disease) may lead to increasing frailty, increasing dependence on the support of others, and fewer opportunities to sustain mental effort. From this standpoint, it is possible to envisage some physical changes being transformed by personality traits into stressors with which the ageing brain copes with reduced efficiency [11]. Stress responses to the physical changes listed earlier appear greater in amplitude and return to baseline (prestressor) levels much more slowly.

The consequences for the individual are often interpreted as placing that individual somewhere along the spectrum melding cognitive ageing with late onset dementias. But this may be an oversimplification. The ageing individual has the opportunity across the life course to acquire multiple self-images, viewing himself or herself quite differently in the various roles of lover, parent, friend, work-mate, and so on. The capacity to sustain an integrated overview of these self-images is affected by mood states and recent stressful experiences such that the same individual may change in the self-image in light of evidence that challenges the belief that he or she is, for example, competent, kind, or helpful. This achievement of a general sense of self is one of the important milestones of adulthood and the threat to its complex integration posed by the ageing brain may convince an individual of his or her powerlessness in the face of ageing and prejudice the view of the future.

Older persons have thus acquired, through personal development and adult maturation, not only a general sense of self but also a working understanding of how people relate to them as individuals and to each other. These general rules are complex but allow older persons to have some certainty about the predictability of the behaviour of others and how it adheres to their own ideas about rules. This type of intuitive understanding is threatened by ageing processes. Ageing challenges the integrity of the self and triggers maladaptive behaviours. Intelligence is but one weapon in the armoury available to blunt the impact of ageing and to slow progression to dementia.

Ageing threatens the structure of the mature personality and is an important disintegrative influence. The maintenance of accurate interpersonal boundaries is a major maturational task in old age when the burden of age-related pathologies impairs sensory information (hearing, vision, and balance) and the confusion created by the fear of losing a personal identity and metamorphosing into someone incapable of independent existence. These processes should be viewed dynamically. The presumption throughout adult life is that the general attributes of an individual's personality remain stable and resist change. As a rule, the intellectual traits are the most stable. Neuroticism increases over the life span as do agreeableness and conscientiousness. However, there are slight declines in extraversion and openness to experience. These personality traits are first viewed as changing little except for some 'mellowing'. Later, as avoidance of uncertainty and ambiguity takes precedence, the old person is seen as having become 'rigid' and preoccupied with 'orderliness' and 'sameness'.

The Scottish Mental Surveys

In 1932 and again in 1947, the Scottish Council for Research in Education undertook two unique surveys [12]. They recruited on each occasion about 95% of eligible school children born in 1921 or 1936 and who were at school on 1 June 1932 or 4 June 1947, respectively. About one hundred sixty thousand children were included in these two surveys that remain unique in the field of educational psychology as the most comprehensive studies of their type. No other nation has attempted to obtain similar data. The IQ test was known as the Moray House Test (number 12) and, in representative samples of one hundred children, it correlated well with the Stamford Binet Test (correlation coefficient = 0.8).

These data provide valid estimates of childhood intelligence. Studies in Aberdeen from 1997 and in Edinburgh from 2000 have shown that the trait of childhood intelligence is very stable over the life course [13]. Repeat testing using the same measures of mental ability showed strong continuity between mental ability test scores for participants aged eleven and seventy-eight years. In Aberdeen ($n = 101$) and Lothian ($n = 500$) sample correlations were 0.68.

In studies of cognitive ageing, the availability of large numbers of childhood mental ability scores for boys and girls possesses many advantages. In terms of the three principles set out at the beginning of this chapter, the mental ability scores provide a baseline against which subsequent cognitive change can be compared. Importantly, simple mathematical models of cognitive variation in old age can first take account of the contribution of childhood intelligence and then test specific hypotheses concerning additional contributions made by putative risk or protective factors encountered at any point in the life span. Childhood mental ability might be a useful proxy for the cognitive reserve available in late life to withstand the burden of brain ageing or neurodegenerative pathologies.

In Aberdeen, longitudinal study measures are intensive and extensive. There are measures of mental speed using the digit symbol subtest, verbal memory using the auditory verbal learning test, and spatial ability using the block design subtest (all from the Weschler Adult Intelligence Scale). A simple test of divergent thinking is provided by the Uses for Objects Test. In addition, general health and physiological integrity can be assessed from cardiorespiratory function (blood pressure, pulse, forced expiratory volume, and ECG), locomotor function using walk time and balance, and selected anthropometric measures (height, weight, and girth). Personality is readily measured using the NEO-FF Personality Scale, mood and anxiety using the Hospital Anxiety Depression scale, and quality of life using SF36 and the Structured Evaluation Inventory for Quality of Life (SEIQoL). Selected biological measures are included, including self-reported frequency of intake of major food groups and fasted blood micronutrient concentrations, together with molecular genetic examination of retained DNA. Environmental and occupational exposures can be rated using an occupational matrix. About 50% of volunteers have volunteered for repeated brain MRI investigation. These MRI measures have been applied at intervals of about fifteen months in the 1921 birth sample from age seventy-seven years onwards and at intervals of two years in the 1936 cohort from age sixty-four onwards.

This work has yielded a rich and diverse database that provides a useful account of trajectories of cognitive ageing in an unselected, nonclinical volunteer sample. All individuals were living independently in the community and at recruitment were without dementia.

Major risk factors

An increased risk of cognitive decline in later life has been associated with female sex, limited educational attainments, and lower childhood mental ability [14]. The contribution of personality traits has also been examined but no consensus exists concerning the relative contributions of each of these risk factors.

Retention of cognitive function in old age is important and a possible contributor to ageing well. When cognitive decline is greater than expected, this predicts progression to dementia and sometimes premature death. Obviously, factors that contribute to differences in rates of cognitive ageing are relevant to understanding choices of preventive measure and the role of causal pathologies. The concept of cognitive reserve has been used to explain some of the individual variation [15]. Long-term studies of those at risk of dementia for reasons of age suggests that early education, adult occupation, a linguistic ability in youth, general health, leisure pursuits, and childhood intelligence may be important [16].

Molecular genetic studies

There are important genetic influences on the diseases of late life. These conditions are major worldwide causes of death and disability. Whilst these diseases are age related, it is by no means clear whether they are age dependent. This is of causal importance, is relevant to understanding cognitive ageing, and may help identify possible gene–environment interactions. If some age-related diseases are shown to be age dependent, then those genes that determine individual differences in rates of ageing might prove relevant to the causal pathways leading to cognitive ageing. So far, few genes that contribute in this way to human ageing are known with certainty, but studies from comparative biology suggest that 'ageing genes' have been conserved in evolution and some are involved in the regulation of energy production [13]. Cognitive ageing genes might, therefore, comprise a complex array of diverse genetic influences acting to increase the risk of developing cognitive ageing and potentially progressing to dementia (Table 6.1).

There are many important genetic influences on cognitive development [14], and it is likely that comparable genetic factors contribute to individual differences in rates of cognitive ageing. At the most obvious level, these genes might include those [15] already known to be involved in Alzheimer's disease (Table 6.2). But whilst these genes are of great importance in dementias with onset before age sixty-five years, they account for much fewer than 5% of late onset dementias. Genes other than the Alzheimer's genes are involved.

The search for these latter contributions illustrates the second of the key principles of ageing research set out previously. Genetic polymorphisms are stable traits that may be associated with childhood IQ, late life cognitive status, or both. We have established that about 50% of cognitive ability in late life is attributable to childhood intelligence ('trait intelligence'), so

Table 6.1 Potential Cognitive Ageing Gene Domains

A	Genes that determine rates of ageing cause faster ageing and accelerate risk of age-dependent disorder
B	Genes that reduce survival because they act early in life to increase risk of childhood onset of fatal disease (e.g., cystic fibrosis); censoring of at-risk population so gene frequency is reduced in late life
C	Genes that convey reproductive advantage in early adulthood but increase susceptibility to late adult onset disease; censoring as B above
D	Genes that increase susceptibility to age-related illnesses (e.g., APOEe4 and vascular or Alzheimer's diseases)
E	Genes that reduce the risk of age-related disease by reducing rates of ageing and risk of specific disorders that are common causes of death (e.g., stroke, heart disease, some cancers)

Table 6.2 Genes and Alzheimer's Disease (AD)

Early onset familial AD		Late onset familial AD	Late onset sporadic AD
Presenilin 1 gene Chromosome 14 Age 25–60	Amyloid precursor protein (APP) gene Chromosome 21 Age 40–65	Presenilin 2 gene Chromosome 1 Age 45–84	APOEe4 allele Chromosome 19 Age >50

Source: Adapted from Thomson, P.A. et al., *Neurosci Lett*, 389, 41, 2005.

genetic associations with late life cognitive status could be determined by primary associations with childhood IQ. Table 6.3 illustrates our approach to this problem and shows that some polymorphisms are linked to childhood IQ and some to late life cognitive status after adjustment for childhood IQ (i.e., these associations are between specific genetic polymorphisms and late life cognition and are not attributable to trait intelligence).

Nutritional studies

Outside the settings of supported and residential care, most old people are free to make varied choices about the food they eat. Their preferences are influenced, amongst other things, by access to food outlets (especially for fresh foods), their ability to follow food cooking or preparation instructions,

Table 6.3 Genetic Polymorphisms, Childhood Intelligence, and Cognitive Ageing

Gene	N	Associated with childhood IQ?	Associated with mental ability age 79 yrs (after adjustment for childhood IQ)?	Ref.
APOEe4	462	No	Yes	16
APOEe4	462	No	Yes, verbal ability	17
ACE	536	No	No	18
MTHFR	536	No	No	18
DISC1	425	No	Yes, general ability	19
Nicastrin	462	Yes	No	20
LTF	417	No	No	21
PRNP	417	No	Yes	21
KLOTHO	464	Yes	Yes	22
COMT	460	No	Yes, verbal memory	23
HSD11B1	194	No	No	24
BDNF	904	No	Yes	25

Acronyms:
APOE = apolipoprotein E; ACE = angiotensin converting enzyme, MTHFR = methionine tetra hydro folate reductase; DISC1 = disrupted in schizophrenia 1; LTF = lactotransferrin; PRNP = prion protein; COMT = catechol-ortho-methyl-transferase; HSD11B1 = 11beta-hydroxysteroid dehydrogenase type 1; BDNF = brain-derived neurotrophic factor

their general physical and mental health, and the social context in which food is to be consumed. Each of these influences can, in turn, be modified by physical, sensory, or cognitive disabilities, sometimes acting in concert.

In the Aberdeen follow-up of the Scottish Mental Surveys, our approach to understanding possible associations between nutritional status and cognitive ageing was divided into observational studies on blood micronutrient concentrations (including homocysteine) and self-reported intake of foodstuffs, including food supplements with, when possible, blood biomarker measurements. The first of these studies [26] measured fasted blood concentrations of plasma and erythrocyte folate, vitamin B_{12}, and homocysteine. In 1999 and 2000, we examined two samples of older people, one born in 1921 (n = 199) and the other born in 1936 (n = 149). Both had completed the same mental ability test when they were aged about eleven years and were recruited in Aberdeen to a longitudinal study of brain ageing and health.

Plasma homocysteine was significantly higher in volunteers born in 1921 than in those born in 1936. Cognitive function test scores were higher in the younger volunteers than in the older, in whom there were positive correlations between folate/B_{12} and cognitive tests and negative correlations between homocysteine and cognitive tests. In the younger subjects, folate was positively correlated with spatial ability. After adjusting both sets (younger and older) of cognitive test scores for childhood intelligence, partial correlations between homocysteine or B_{12} and cognitive test scores were maintained in the same direction and strengthened. We argued that in late old age (the subjects born in 1921), there are strong relationships between homocysteine, vitamin B_{12}/folate, and cognitive function, where homocysteine accounted for about 8% of the variance in cognitive test scores. These relationships were not seen in early old age (the subjects born in 1936), when there may be opportunities to slow later age-related cognitive decline using supplements of B_{12}/folate.

These relationships were explored further in a structural brain MRI study of the older subjects [27]. Here, plasma homocysteine and cholesterol were found associated with brain shrinkage (atrophy) whereas plasma vitamin C was associated with retention of brain grey matter. These findings were interpreted conservatively as providing support for a possible role of vascular risk factors in brain ageing and age-related cognitive decline.

The use of dietary supplements (DS) was examined in a subset of 176 subjects drawn from the sample born in 1921 [28]. DS users did not differ from DS nonusers in years of education, socioeconomic status, or measures of cardiorespiratory function. DS use was more frequent in those with higher childhood IQ, in women than in men, in those of lower BMI, and in those taking fewer prescribed medications. Intake of foodstuffs (as assessed by food frequency from the MONICA surveys) showed that usual diet did not differ between DS users and DS nonusers but that there were differences in blood micronutrient concentrations. DS users had higher vitamin C and alpha-carotene, and lower gamma tocopherol and homocysteine concentrations than those in non DS users.

Table 6.4 Cognitive Test Scores[a] by Category of Food Supplement Use in 266
Community Residents from the 1936 Scottish Mental Survey

Cognitive test	Food supplement category				Statistical significance
	Nonuser n = 229	Fish oil n = 72	Vitamins n = 29	Other n = 20	
IQ age 11 yrs	99.6 ± 15.1	103.9 ± 14.4	106.1 ± 13.9	101.6 ± 11.9	Not significant
IQ age 64/65 yrs	98.4 ± 14.9	104.1 ± 14.9[b]	107.2 ± 17.2[b]	105.2 ± 11.7[b]	$p < 0.01$
Digit symbol test	42.0 ± 11.7	47.5 ± 11.0[c]	50.6 ± 12.5[c]	51.2 ± 9.9[c]	$p < 0.001$

[a] Mean + sd

[b] Significantly greater than nonusers.

[c] Significantly greater than nonusers before and after adjustment for IQ age eleven years.

We approached the study of DS use in the 1936 sample from a different standpoint [29]. First, we classified DS users by choice of principal supplement (fish oil, vitamin preparation, or 'other') and compared current cognitive and childhood IQ test scores. Although childhood IQ did not differ between DS category, there were differences in scores on current cognitive tests (age sixty-four and sixty-five years) (Table 6.4). However, after adjusting current cognitive scores for childhood IQ, only performance on the digit symbol test (measuring mental speed and attention) remained significantly different between categories of DS use or between DS users and DS nonusers. In a case-control study nested in the larger sample, erythrocyte membrane n-3 fatty acid content was higher in fish oil supplement users than in nonusers. After adjustment for childhood IQ, a raised ratio of docosahexaenoic acid (an n-3 fatty acid found mostly in fish) to arachidonic acid (an n-6 fatty acid) was associated with better cognitive function in early old age.

These studies suggested to us that the use of childhood IQ as a baseline from which to estimate lifelong cognitive variation was valid and could be extended to studies in community-resident volunteers using the methods of nutritional epidemiology. We also began to suspect that childhood intelligence was exerting other indirect influence on health status in late life, perhaps through the acquisition not only of healthy eating habits but also of other health-related behaviours.

Health-related behaviours

Childhood intelligence could potentially prove relevant to understanding the association between low social class and inequalities in health that persist across the life course extending into old age. We considered a number of possible pathways along which such a modifying effect might be exerted, starting with the likely influence of childhood IQ on the acquisition of health-related behaviours. Smoking is one such behaviour: It is a hazardous activity related to poor respiratory and vascular health and, through its association with cerebrovascular disease and stroke, possibly linked to progressive age-related cognitive decline and progress to dementia.

First, in the Aberdeen sample born in 1936, we examined whether smoking was a risk factor for relative cognitive decline from age eleven to sixty-four years [30]. We sought to allow for the effects of coexisting heart disease, hypertension, poor lung function, and lower socioeconomic status. Current smokers had lower cognitive test scores than nonsmokers at age sixty-four and sixty-five years. We re-examined these questions in a second independent sample [31]. Here, structural equation models suggested that childhood IQ was not directly associated with smoking but acted through mechanisms associated with poverty. Each standard deviation (i.e., fifteen points) IQ disadvantage increased by about 21% the risk of having a smoking-related hospital admission, cancer, or death during a twenty-five-year follow-up period. These studies raised more general questions concerning the mechanisms by which lower childhood IQ could be linked in the Aberdeen studies to greater than expected mortality [2], which we explored as follows.

The Scottish Mental Surveys were linked to the MIDSPAN studies undertaken in Renfrew and Paisley, Scotland, in the 1970s. These studies were designed to detect major risk factors for vascular disease in a population known to have amongst the highest worldwide incidence rates for vascular disease. We matched 938 individuals, born in 1921, from the MIDSPAN studies with the Scottish 1932 Mental Survey [32]. Morbidity related to cancer, hospital admissions, and all-cause mortality were related to childhood IQ, deprivation, and socioeconomic status. As shown earlier, the risk of dying in the twenty-five-year follow-up period was 17% higher for each standard deviation disadvantage in childhood IQ. Once adjustment was made for social class and deprivation, this increase was reduced to about 12%. Cause-specific mortality or cancer incidence risk was higher with decreasing IQ for lung cancer. These data supported the general conclusion that childhood IQ shares with social class some but not all of the mechanisms linking low social class with poor health in later life.

However, the exact mechanisms of this association were unclear. First, we examined the role of hypertension in the preceding sample of 938 individuals [33]. Midlife systolic and diastolic hypertension, childhood intelligence, sex, height, and weight were investigated. For each standard deviation increase in childhood IQ, there was a 3.2-mmHg decrease in diastolic blood pressure after adjustment for age, sex, social class, and body mass index. We concluded that previously reported associations between hypertension and impaired cognitive function in late life were in part determined by differences in childhood IQ. The specific association between childhood IQ and lung function and cardiovascular risk factors was further analysed in this sample [34]. With each standard deviation decrease in childhood IQ, there was an increased risk before age sixty-five years of cerebrovascular disease (relative risk [RR] = 1.11; 95% confidence interval [CI] = 1.01–1.23) and coronary heart disease (RR = 1.16; 95% CI = 1.03–1.32), but not stroke (RR = 1.10; 95% CI = 0.88–1.36). Blood pressure, height, respiratory function, and smoking were linked with cerebrovascular events. There were slight reductions in cerebrovascular disease risk after adjustment for childhood IQ.

Follow-up studies of the Scottish mental surveys have established childhood IQ as a novel risk factor for vascular disease in adult life and this may be related to a reported significant increase in dementia incidence observed in individuals with low average IQ [35]. When childhood IQ is introduced into statistical models of the association between low social class and increased mortality, the association is much, but not completely, reduced. The proposition that childhood intelligence is the 'epidemiologist's elusive fundamental cause of social class inequalities in health' is therefore not supported by these studies [36].

Conclusions

The Scottish Mental Surveys were undertaken to determine the educational needs of two generations of Scottish children. They have proven to be an invaluable resource in the investigation of individual differences in the development of cognitive abilities across the life course and in understanding some genetic and nutritional sources of these differences. The survivors of the original surveys have now been recruited into longitudinal studies of brain ageing and health and, perhaps unexpectedly, they are making fresh and sometimes novel contributions to the study of ageing.

Some of these volunteers are 'ageing well' and are doing so for a great diversity of reasons. Amongst these is the significant role played by their initial, childhood intelligence. These measures have provided not only a useful baseline from which to estimate change but also a gateway into better understanding of the geography of cognitive ageing and dementia. It is now possible to place in that landscape some key features, including choices to eat a healthy diet, judicious use of food supplements, not smoking, frequent health checks, and reduction of exposure to risk of vascular disease, and so to navigate a healthy course to ageing well and successfully.

References

1. Hadley, E.C. et al. Genetic epidemiologic studies on age-specified traits. *Am J Epidemiol*, 152, 1003, 2000.
2. Whalley, L.J. and Deary, I.J. Longitudinal cohort study of childhood IQ and survival up to age 76. *BMJ*, 322, 819, 2001.
3. Hart, C.L. et al. Childhood IQ, social class, deprivation, and their relationships with mortality and morbidity risk in later life: Prospective observational study linking the Scottish Mental Survey 1932 and the Midspan studies. *Psychosom Med*, 65, 877, 2003.

4. Deary, I.J. et al. The impact of childhood intelligence on later life: Following up the Scottish mental surveys of 1932 and 1947. *J Pers Soc Psychol*, 86, 130, 2004.

5. Stern, Y. What is cognitive reserve? Theory and research application of the reserve concept. *J Int Neuropsychol Soc*, 8, 448, 2002.

6. Whalley, L.J., Dick, F.D., and McNeill, G. A life-course approach to the aetiology of late-onset dementias. *Lancet Neurol*, 5, 87, 2006.

7. de Magalhaes, J.P. and Sandberg, A. Cognitive aging as an extension of brain development: A model linking learning, brain plasticity, and neurodegeneration. *Mech Ageing Dev*, 126, 1026, 2005.

8. Arendt, T. Alzheimerís disease as a disorder of dynamic brain self-organization. *Prog Brain Res*, 147, 355, 2005.

9. Fratiglioni, L., Paillard-Borg, S., and Winblad, B. An integrated and socially integrated lifestyle in late life might protect against dementia. *Lancet Neurol*, 3, 343, 2004.

10. Bennett, D.A. et al., The effect of social networks on the relation between Alzheimer's disease pathology and level of cognitive function in old people: A longitudinal cohort study. *Lancet Neurol*, 5, 87, 2006.

11. Whalley, L., *The Ageing Brain*. Phoenix, London, 88–112, 2002.

12. Deary, I.J. et al. The stability of individual differences in mental ability from childhood to old age: Follow-up of the 1932 Scottish mental survey. *Intelligence*, 28, 49, 2000.

13. Warner, H.R. Longevity genes: From primitive organisms to humans. *Mech Ageing Dev*, 126, 235, 2005.

14. Deary, I.J. et al. Searching for genetic influences on normal cognitive ageing. *Trends Cogn Sci*, 8, 178, 2004.

15. Bertram, L. and Tanzi, R.E. Alzheimer's disease: One disorder, too many genes? *Hum Mol Genet*, 13, R135, sp. iss., 1, 2004.

16. Deary, I.J. et al. Cognitive change and the APOE epsilon 4 allele. *Nature*, 418, 932, 2002.

17. Deary, I.J. et al. Apolipoprotein e gene variability and cognitive functions at age 79: A follow-up of the Scottish mental survey of 1932. *Psychol Aging*, 19, 36, 2004.

18. Visscher, P.M. et al. Lack of association between polymorphisms in angiotensin-converting enzyme and methylenetetrahydrofolate reductase genes and normal cognitive ageing in humans. *Neurosci Lett*, 347, 175, 2003.

19. Thomson, P.A. et al. Association between genotype at an exonic SNP in DISC1 and normal cognitive aging. *Neurosci Lett*, 389, 41, 2005.

20. Deary, I.J. et al. Nicastrin gene polymorphisms, cognitive ability level and cognitive ageing. *Neurosci Lett*, 373, 110, 2005.

21. Kachiwala, S.J. et al. Genetic influences on oxidative stress and their association with normal cognitive ageing. *Neurosci Lett*, 386, 116, 2005.

22. Deary, I.J., Harris, S.E., Fox, H.C., Hayward, C., Wright, A.F., Starr, J.M., and Whalley, L.J. KLOTHO genotype and cognitive ability in childhood and old age in the same individuals. *Neurosci Lett*, 378, 22, 2005.

23. Harris, S.E., Wright, A.F., Hayward, C., Starr, J.M., Whalley, L.J., and Deary, I.J. The functional COMT polymorphism, Val 158 Met, is associated with logical memory and the personality trait intellect/imagination in a cohort of healthy 79-year-olds. *Neurosci Lett*, 385, 1, 2005.

24. Deary, I.J. Polymorphisms in the gene encoding 11B-hydroxysteroid dehydrogenase type 1 (HSD11B1) and lifetime cognitive change. *Neurosci Lett*, 393, 74, 2006.

25. Harris, S.E. et al. The brain-derived neurotrophic factor Val66Met polymorphism is associated with age-related change in reasoning skills. *Mol Psychiatry*, 11, 505, 2006.

26. Duthie, S.J. et al. Homocysteine, B vitamin status, and cognitive function in the elderly. *Am J Clin Nutr*, 75, 908, 2002.

27. Whalley, L.J. et al. Plasma vitamin C, cholesterol and homocysteine are associated with grey matter volume determined by MRI in nondemented old people. *Neurosci Lett*, 341, 173, 2003.

28. Whalley, L.J. Dietary supplement use in old age: Associations with childhood IQ, current cognition and health. *Int J Geriatr Psychiatry*, 18, 769, 2003.

29. Whalley, L.J. et al. Cognitive aging, childhood intelligence, and the use of food supplements: possible involvement of n-3 fatty acids. *Am J Clin Nutr*, 80, 1650, 2004.

30. Whalley, L.J. et al. Childhood IQ, smoking, and cognitive change from age 11 to 64 years. *Addict Behav*, 30, 77, 2005.

31. Taylor, M.D. et al. Childhood IQ and social factors on smoking behaviour, lung function and smoking-related outcomes in adulthood: Linking the Scottish Mental Survey 1932 and the Midspan studies. *Br J Health Psychol*, 10, 399, 2005.

32. Hart, C.L. et al. Childhood IQ and all-cause mortality before and after age 65: Prospective observational study linking the Scottish Mental Survey 1932 and the Midspan studies. *Br J Health Psychol*, 10, 153, 2005.

33. Starr, J.M. et al. Childhood mental ability and blood pressure at midlife: Linking the Scottish Mental Survey 1932 and the Midspan studies. *J Hypertens*, 22, 893, 2004.

34. Hart, C.L. et al. Childhood IQ and cardiovascular disease in adulthood: Prospective observational study linking the Scottish Mental Survey 1932 and the Midspan studies. *Soc Sci Med*, 59, 2131, 2004.

35. Whalley, L.J. et al. Childhood mental ability and dementia. *Neurology*, 55, 1455, 2000.

36. Batty, G.D. et al. Does IQ explain socioeconomic inequalities in health? Evidence from a population-based cohort study in the west of Scotland. *BMJ*, 332, 580, 2006.

chapter seven

Health inequalities in old age in Britain

Elizabeth Breeze

Contents

Why study inequalities in old age?...67
Theories relating socioeconomic position to variation in health.................68
Findings...70
    Source data..70
    Socioeconomic position in middle age affects health status
        in old age...70
    Does socioeconomic position still have an influence in old age? 75
        Longitudinal studies within old age..75
        Transitions in socioeconomic status in late middle age
            or early old age and subsequent quality of
            life and mortality...76
Policy implications 78
References...80

Why study inequalities in old age?

By the time people reach old age, it might be considered too late to act concerning health inequalities. However, the growing numbers and percentages of older people mean that policies to cater for older age are no longer a minor consideration in budgeting. At the time of the Sutherland Commission in 1999, it was estimated that '2.2% of taxes from earnings, pensions and investments is spent on long-term care in residential settings and in people's homes' [1]. In the National Service Framework, it was stated that 'at any one time, older people occupy around two-thirds of hospital beds' [2].

The health inequalities of concern in this chapter are 'differences in prevalence or incidence of health problems between individual people of higher and lower socioeconomic status' [3]. The purpose of identifying health inequalities is to open the way for consideration of how they can be reduced. Woodward and Kawachi [4] summarise four arguments for reducing health inequalities: Inequalities are unfair (moral argument); they affect everyone (self-interest argument); they are avoidable; and they can be reduced cost effectively.

Many researchers remark on the variability in health, fitness, and well-being of people in their seventies and beyond [5,6] and that some people move from disabled to able state even in old age [7–9]. Declining mean levels of physical function with age conceal a wide variety of individual trajectories [10]. A motivation for research into health inequalities is the knowledge that health problems are not automatic companions of old age. People do not usually choose relative disadvantage with respect to education, income, housing, and other aspects of living conditions. These living conditions influence health. Where possible, we should seek the removal of society-wide barriers to good health, such as lack of material or educational resources, or find ways of compensating for them.

Theories relating socioeconomic position to variation in health

The Black Report, commissioned by the U.K. Department of Health in 1977 to look at health differences between social classes, listed four theoretical approaches to explanations of inequalities [11]. The first refutes inequality in two ways, one claiming it is because the least healthy are left in the diminishing group of unskilled jobs and the other that it is not class per se that matters but the composition of the class [12]. A second approach attributes observed differences to selective mobility whereby the most vulnerable drift downwards or are left behind in the lower group and the sturdiest move upwards (reverse causation or health selection). Health selection [13] during working life can serve to constrain rather than extend differentials because people who move categories may have chances of poor health that are intermediate between that of the group they left and that of the group they joined [14,15]. Reverse causation is not now thought to account for major class differentials [16].

The third approach, a materialist or structuralist explanation, gives some credit to direct effects of absolute poverty, but is more concerned with the way in which society is structured to limit opportunities for some. The fourth approach emphasises individual behaviour in a cultural context (e.g., higher percentages of people in manual classes smoking, having a poor diet, and taking little exercise).

Several other theories have been put forward. One group of arguments refers to the practical opportunities denied to people in a worse socioeconomic position and direct effects of exposure to hazards that are part of being in a particular socioeconomic position [17]. A second type of argument takes psychosocial stress to be a major pathway for poor health and poverty. Two pathways to ill health are proposed [18]: a direct one whereby chronic stress causes changes to the neuroendocrine, metabolic, and immune systems [19] and an indirect one via adoption of risky behaviours. The psychosocial theory of health damage is linked to the context in which people live to produce the hypothesis that being in an area of marked income inequality creates stresses and hence poorer health. This theory sets out to answer why some societies (rather than individuals) are healthier than others. Wilkinson argues that greater income inequality reduces social cohesion in poorer neighbourhoods and also leads to greater within-family stress [20].

Many of these theories are woven together in the life-course approach, which suggests that 'throughout the life course exposures or insults gradually accumulate through episodes of illness, adverse environmental conditions and behaviours, increasing the risk of chronic disease and mortality' [21]. Early life circumstances may have direct effects on health or indirect effects via opportunities and lifestyle that in turn cause health problems. Different pathways are proposed—for example, a predominantly biologically determined one starting with early nutrition or repeated infection, and a predominantly socially and economically determined one of limited or plentiful opportunities for employment or a healthy lifestyle. Health-related behaviour is seldom chosen completely freely; it is heavily influenced by social status and cultural milieu [18]. The relative importance of different periods of life to different health conditions may vary. Davey Smith observed that behaviour risk factors are more dependent on adulthood social position than parental social class, so their modification is 'dependent on the presence of social circumstances required for maintaining favourable health-related behaviours' [22].

An implication of most of the theories is that health inequalities will not be reduced substantially by expecting individuals to alter their lifestyles in a vacuum and that provision of health services alone would not suffice.

There are many measures of socioeconomic position, some leaning towards material influences, others to status and stress [23,24]. Income and wealth reflect ability to buy a healthy life but also status; education enhances life's opportunities to gain material resources but also to make the best use of the services society has to offer; housing tenure can be related directly to hazards (e.g., living in polluted areas) but also to status and material circumstances. Finally, the current U.K. socioeconomic classification of jobs is based on the nature of the contract people have, with underlying concepts of demand–control and effort–reward balances. The former social class classification was meant to reflect status; the details lacked a clear conceptual framework yet it was correlated with many health and illness experiences.

Findings

Source data

The findings quoted here come from three studies and are enhanced by comparisons with other studies. The first study used the census-based Longitudinal Study (LS) to look at health outcomes in 1991 in relation to socioeconomic positions in 1971 and 1981 [25,26]. The Longitudinal Study population used in these analyses comprises 1% of people from the 1971 British Census, who have been tracked through subsequent censuses and vital events. The second study used a resurvey of the first cohort of male London civil servants (Whitehall Study) to model self-reported health in the late 1990s, nearly thirty years after the original screening in the late 1960s [27,28]. The third study analysed quality of life, measured by four dimensions of the Sickness Impact Profile [29] and the Philadelphia Geriatric Morale Scale [30,31]. The sample for the third study came from the MRC Trial of the Assessment and Management of People aged seventy-five years and over in Britain (MRC Study) and was derived from a sample of fifty-three general practices [32].

Socioeconomic position in middle age affects health status in old age

Data from the Longitudinal Study and the Whitehall Study demonstrate that there are long-lasting effects of socioeconomic position in midlife on a variety of health outcomes in old age. This effect was present for mortality and being in an institution as well as to quality of life measures such as self-rated health and daily functioning. In each case, the chances of poor outcomes were worse if a person had two or more disadvantages rather than one (for example, lack of car and being in a rented home, or lower employment grade and being in a rented home). This is of particular concern because the poor health outcomes in the Whitehall Study identified minority groups (defined as roughly 10% of the sample) who performed *considerably* worse on the health indicators than the rest of the cohort. Using a cumulative socioeconomic index on the Whitehall Study, it was clear that prevalences of poor outcomes vary widely according to socioeconomic circumstances (Figures 7.1a through 7.1d). For example, for poor physical performance, the predicted prevalence ranges from 9% with no socioeconomic disadvantage to 35% with two disadvantages for the oldest age group (age eighty years or over at resurvey).

The Whitehall data cover a restricted population of males in secure employment with a good pension scheme and yet they too demonstrate substantial variability in health status in old age according to socioeconomic status. The LS population was larger, more heterogeneous, and more representative, but used fairly crude socioeconomic classifications; more refined measures may have revealed a greater degree of inequality. The strength of the findings is surprising in the context of selective survival. In the LS only one third of the younger cohort of men and half of younger women (aged

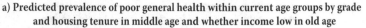

a) Predicted prevalence of poor general health within current age groups by grade and housing tenure in middle age and whether income low in old age

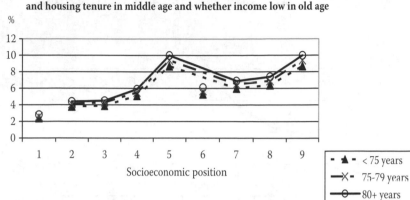

b) Predicted prevalence of poor mental health within current age groups by grade and housing tenure in middle age and whether income low in old age

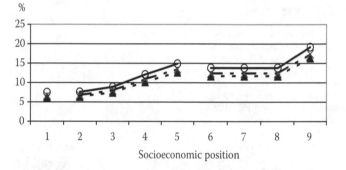

c) Predicted prevalence of poor physical performance within current age groups by grade and housing tenure in middle age and whether income low in old age

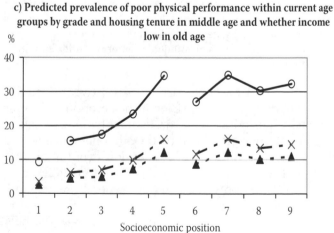

Figure 7.1

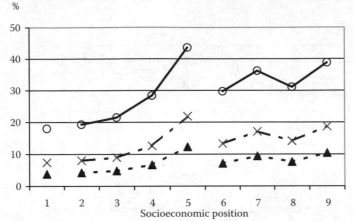

d) **Predicted prevalence of disability within current age groups by grade and housing tenure in middle age and whether income low in old age**

General key for socioeconomic position:
1= Administrative
2 = Professional/executive, owner-occupier, not low income
3= Professional/executive, renter, not low income
4 = Professional/executive, owner-occupier, low income
5= Professional/executive, renter, low income
6 = Clerical/manual, owner-occupier, not low income
7= Clerical/manual, renter, not low income
8 = Clerical/manual, owner-occupier, low income
9= Clerical/manual, renter, low income

Figure 7.1 Predicted prevalence of poor self-reported outcomes in 1997–1998 by age and cumulative index of socioeconomic position: Whitehall Study. General key for socioeconomic position: 1 = administrative; 2 = professional/executive, owner occupier, not low income; 3 = professional/executive, renter, not low income; 4 = professional/executive, owner occupier, low income; 5 = professional/executive, renter, low income; 6 = clerical/manual, owner occupier, not low income; 7 = clerical/manual, renter, not low income; 8 = clerical/manual, owner occupier, low income; 9 = clerical/manual, renter, low income.

fifty-five to sixty-four years at baseline) had survived twenty years in the community. It would not have been surprising if socioeconomic differentials had evened out over this period because, on the one hand, the sickest had died or moved into long-term care whilst, on the other hand, some forms of long-standing illness were becoming fairly common even amongst those who started healthy and socioeconomically advantaged in 1971.

In the Whitehall study, not only was survival generally worse in lower grades (18% of the original cohort participating in the resurvey compared with over 40% of others) but also, within the grades, it was the healthier who survived. For example, 26% of the full cohort of clerical and manual staff had evidence of heart disease at baseline but only 14% of survivors. Yet these 'healthier' people from the manual grades still had worse health than the survivors from the higher grades.

This evidence of the continued influence on morbidity of socioeconomic position from midlife into old age in Britain suggests that action to counter socioeconomic disadvantage in middle age might continue to show benefits well into old age. Hitherto, only one analysis had looked at health differentials persisting twenty or more years—that of mortality of the Whitehall cohort [33]. LS analyses of mortality by age at death over shorter follow-up periods had led to the conclusion that household socioeconomic measures were stronger discriminators than individual ones (own social class) and this was clear also in our long-term results, although social class may have been poorly classified because it was collected retrospectively, and the group of unclassified women are likely to be heterogeneous. In a study of American men, the longest held occupation influenced mortality over a follow-up period of approximately seventeen years after the subjects reached the age of fifty-five years [34]. Olausson [35] did not find a clear-cut trend in mortality by social class in middle age in Sweden but exclusion of the unemployed probably reduced the differentials.

Evidence of long-term socioeconomic effects on functioning comes from the United States and Sweden. U.S. studies with follow-up of twenty years or more include the Alameda cohort with respect to income [36] and education [37], the Honolulu cohort with respect to occupation [38], and the Charleston cohort with respect to education (amongst white women only) [39]. In Sweden, the less educated were more likely, and white collar workers less likely, to have limitations in activities of daily living and in mobility twenty years after baseline, although there was not a difference by occupational class for self-rated health and results were weaker for women [40–42].

As well as longitudinal studies, cross-sectional studies can give some backing to continuing relevance of socioeconomic position in middle age for health status in old age, if they use socioeconomic measures that were determined by middle age. In the MRC Study it was clear that those who had been in local authority accommodation most of their adult lives or in the manual occupational classes were at greater risk of poor quality of life (Table 7.1). Other cross-sectional studies in Britain found associations between social class and limiting long-term illness, self-rated health, psychosocial well-being, and disability [43–47]. In contrast, in the Health and Lifestyle Study, differences in functioning by social class were small amongst people aged seventy years and over, although differences remained for self-reported illness [44]. The balance of evidence from Britain, the United States [48], and Europe [49–51] is in favour of continued adverse influence of socioeconomic disadvantage in middle age on mortality, on day-to-day functioning, and on perceived health in old age.

Table 7.1 Odds Ratios (ORs) and 95% Confidence Intervals (CIs) for Being in the Worst Quintile of Quality of Life Score by Socioeconomic Position in Midlife[a]

	Home management[b] N = 8,278		Mobility[b] N = 8,277		Body care and management[b] N = 8,279		Social interaction[b] N = 8,275		Morale[c] N = 8,262	
	OR[d]	95% CI	OR[d]	95% CI	OR[d]	95% CI	OR[d]	95% CI	OR[d]	95% CI
Social class[e]										
I/II	1.0		1.0		1.0		1.0		1.0	
IIINM	1.0	(0.8, 1.3)	1.1	(0.9, 1.3)	1.1	(0.9, 1.4)	1.1	(0.9, 1.5)	1.4	(1.1, 1.7)
IIIM	1.5	(1.2, 1.8)	1.4	(1.1, 1.7)	1.4	(1.2, 1.6)	1.4	(1.2, 1.8)	1.5	(1.2, 1.8)
IV/V	1.5	(1.2, 1.9)	1.6	(1.2, 2.0)	1.4	(1.1, 1.8)	1.6	(1.3, 2.0)	1.4	(1.1, 1.7)
AF, NJ, NC[f]	1.8	(1.2, 2.7)	1.7	(1.1, 2.7)	1.4	(1.0, 2.1)	1.7	(1.3, 2.1)	1.0	(0.7, 1.3)
p-value	0.012		0.004		0.010		<0.001		0.007	
Housing tenure most of adult life[e]										
Owner occupied	1.0		1.0		1.0		1.0		1.0	
Local authority[g]	1.5	(1.3, 1.7)	1.6	(1.3, 2.0)	1.7	(1.5, 2.0)	1.4	(1.2, 1.6)	1.5	(1.3, 1.7)
Other	1.3	(1.0, 1.6)	1.2	(1.0, 1.5)	1.3	(1.1, 1.6)	1.2	(1.0, 1.5)	1.2	(1.0, 1.4)
p-value	<0.001		0.001		<0.001		0.001		<0.001	
Car ownership										
Never vs. ever	0.9	(0.8, 1.1)	1.0	(0.8, 1.2)	0.9	(0.8, 1.1)	1.2	(1.0, 1.4)	1.0	(0.9, 1.2)
p-value	0.47		0.85		0.32		0.072		0.93	

a MRC Trial of the Assessment and Management of Older People in the Community 1995–1999.

b From the Sickness Impact Profile.

c From the Philadelphia Geriatric Morale Scale.

d Adjusted for gender, age, marital status, tertiles of area Jarman (deprivation) score, and area standardised mortality ratio.

e Asked retrospectively.

f Armed forces (AF), no job (NJ), not classifiable (NC). For women, the predominant group was 'no job', for men it was armed forces.

g Local authority and housing association.

Does socioeconomic position still have an influence in old age?

There are three ways of addressing this question. First, use longitudinal studies of change in outcome during old age relative to socioeconomic position held at the beginning of the period. Second, it is sometimes possible to surmise a causal sequence from cross-sectional studies describing how health status varies with current socioeconomic position (this approach is not discussed further here). Third and most powerfully, the health impact of changes in socioeconomic position later in life can be studied.

Longitudinal studies within old age

The older cohort of the Longitudinal Study was aged sixty-five to seventy-four years in 1971, and the fact that mortality over the following twenty years was higher for people in rented accommodation and without a car shows that selective survival had not yet removed all socioeconomic differences for those who had attained this age. This cohort was aged eighty-six to ninety-four in 1991 and still demonstrated socioeconomic health inequalities in institutional residence. Limiting long-term illness did not vary so much by socioeconomic position for the very old cohort, although there was a small excess risk for women in rented housing without a car.

Other analyses of the Longitudinal Study reinforced our findings that owner occupiers and/or people with a car had a lower rate of mortality [52–54] even after age sixty-five. In particular, Goldblatt noted that the household measures performed better than social class as predictors of mortality; these could also be seen as measures of current material circumstances. In addition, two of the studies analysed mortality occurring after a time lag during which effects of health selection should have worn off. Salas [55], on the other hand, judged that socioeconomic position appeared to worsen general health but not to the extent of increasing mortality over a four-year period, after adjusting for several intermediate variables and baseline health.

Several longitudinal studies following up people within old age have results consistent with various measures of socioeconomic position having some impact on mortality within old age. In some of these cases, multiple measures contributed independently [56–58], whereas in others they did not [59]. Additional evidence that the impact happened after baseline came from the Longitudinal Study of Aging, in which there was little change in the odds ratios for disability by education or poverty after adjusting for disability at baseline [7].

There is evidence that people with lower socioeconomic position in old age have worse prospects for subsequent self-rated health, mobility, or disability. This applies to self-rated health in Britain [55,60], retention of physical ability or successful ageing in the United States [61,62], and decline in mobility or functioning in the United States [6,7,63,64] and Spain. However, the evidence for health inequalities was not universal, and in North American studies socioeconomic position was not found to be related to successful ageing [65] or to decline in activities of daily living [66] or to onset of self-care problems [6].

Transitions in socioeconomic status in late middle age or early old age and subsequent quality of life and mortality

One of the clearest indications that the influence of socioeconomic factors continues to accumulate into old age is evident when a change in socioeconomic position is followed by a change in quality of life and functioning. Changes in socioeconomic position were not common in the general population, and over a ten-year period about one in nine people changed housing tenure (other than going to an institution) in the LS. It was more common for car availability to change, with over 10% ceasing to have access in this period and 5 or 6% gaining household access to a car. The resurvey of civil servants took place twenty-nine years after screening; between the first screening and leaving the Civil Service, two fifths of the professional/executive staff and over half the clerical/manual staff had risen a category (for some, this would have involved more than one promotion). In the cross-sectional MRC Study, the transitions analysed were changes from living in local authority accommodation during 'most of my adult life' to living in owner-occupation housing in old age and vice versa; the analyses here are restricted to those living alone or with their spouse in old age to reduce the chances of reverse causation. These transitions excluded people who moved to sheltered housing and people in 'other' rental situations and may explain why the percentages were smaller than those reported for the LS.

In the Longitudinal Study changing from an owner-occupying to a renting household carried increased risks of mortality, being in an institution, and having a limiting long-term illness for women aged fifty-five to seventy-four years who made the change during the following ten years. The only exception was that younger women did not have a statistically significant increase in risk of a limiting long-term illness. Amongst men who changed to rented accommodation, the observed risks of these outcomes were generally not statistically significantly raised, but this was partly because of small numbers; the point estimates were as large as those for women in some cases. Losing access to a car was associated more generally with worsened risk of the LS outcomes amongst the younger generation and also of mortality amongst older men. In each case, the risk or odds ratio for this transition group compared to people retaining the socioeconomic advantage, where statistically significant, was of similar magnitude to, or greater than, the equivalent ratio for people who were in the disadvantaged position both in 1971 and in 1981.

In the MRC Study, the change from owner-occupation to social housing (including housing associations) amongst those living alone or with a spouse was also generally associated with greater chance of poor quality of life for this group (Table 7.2). Furthermore, the odds of poor social interaction or morale for those who made the change were similar to those for people who

Table 7.2 Odds Ratios (ORs) and 95% Confidence Intervals (CIs) for Being in the Worst Quintile of Quality of Life Score: Comparing Groups of Respondents Who Changed Housing Tenure with Those Who Did Not: People Living Alone or with Spouse; MRC Study[a,b]

	Home management (N = 8,528)		Mobility (N = 8,526)		Body care and management (N = 8,526)		Social interaction (N = 8,524)		Morale (N = 8,509)	
	OR	95% CI	OR	95% CI	OR	95% CI	OR	95% CI	OR	95% CI
Comparison with source tenure										
Move to social sector vs. stay in owner occupied[c]	1.5	(1.0, 2.4)	1.3	(0.8, 2.1)	2.0	(1.3, 3.1)	1.6	(1.1, 2.4)	1.5	(1.0, 2.3)
Move to 'other' tenure vs. stay in owner occupied[d]	1.6	(1.0, 2.6)	1.4	(0.8, 2.3)	1.4	(0.9, 2.3)	1.3	(0.8, 2.1)	1.4	(0.9, 2.2)
Move to owner occupied vs. stay in social sector	0.8	(0.6, 1.0)	0.9	(0.6, 1.4)	1.0	(0.8, 1.3)	0.6	(0.4, 0.9)	0.8	(0.6, 1.2)
Move to owner occupied vs. stay in 'other' tenure	0.7	(0.4, 1.1)	0.7	(0.5, 1.0)	1.0	(0.7, 1.5)	1.3	(0.9, 1.9)	0.8	(0.5, 1.3)
Comparison with destination tenure										
Move to social sector from owner occupied vs. stay in social sector	0.6	(0.4, 0.9)	0.7	(0.5, 1.0)	0.7	(0.5, 1.0)	0.9	(0.5, 1.4)	1.0	(0.7, 1.4)
Move to owner occupied from social sector vs. stay in owner occupied	1.5	(1.1, 2.1)	1.9	(1.4, 2.5)	2.2	(1.8, 2.8)	1.2	(0.7, 1.4)	1.5	(1.1, 2.0)

a Adjusted for gender, age, marital status, tertiles of Jarman score, and tertiles of SMR.

b All fifteen tenure categories were in one model but odds ratios have been reworked to show variation within category of housing tenure for most of life.

c Move into local authority or housing association housing.

d Move into privately rented housing or rent free (including changes of ownership to ownership by relatives).

had been in social-sector housing in both midlife and old age. However, the confidence intervals were wide. In the Whitehall Study, the professional/ executive staff who had a low income after retirement had higher prevalence of poor health outcomes than those who did not; although it is not known when their income became low, it is quite likely that they had suffered a drop in their socioeconomic position.

There were mixed results for the health status of people who had improved their socioeconomic position. For the most part, the risks of LS outcomes amongst people who had changed from renting to owner-occupation housing were no worse than amongst people who had been in owner occupation housing at both time points. The exceptions could be explained by health selection. A more specific change from local authority housing to owner-occupation housing was considered in the MRC Study. In contrast to the LS, the 'upward' transition appeared to bring no advantage or disadvantage for three of the quality of life dimensions (mobility, self-care, and morale) over those who had been in social-sector housing both in midlife and in old age. The risk of poor home management was reduced for the upward movers but not to the level of people who had been in owner occupation all the time. Social interaction was the only measure for which the chances of poor outcome amongst the upward transition group were similar to those for people in owner occupation at both periods. In the Whitehall Study, a promotion from the lowest category to a higher one reduced the odds of poor mental health, poor physical performance, and disability by 30% or more for people compared with men who stayed in the lowest category.

These analyses of transitions provide a new perspective on socioeconomic factors in old age; only one study found in the literature concentrated on transitions [8]. Unfortunately, the evidence from the three projects analysed in this chapter is more consistent in suggesting negative effects of deterioration in socioeconomic position than positive effects from an improvement. Further research is needed to understand pathways more fully and to see how socioeconomic transitions arise and which ones are most common.

The numbers that changed status in these studies may be relatively small, but there are two messages arising from the results on transitions. First, services that cater for older people should be alert to those whose socioeconomic position is deteriorating. Second is the wider message that socioeconomic position still exerts influence in old age. Even if people attained their current socioeconomic situation partly through earlier experience of health or sickness, that position can in turn have implications for future health.

Policy implications

A major aspect of any policy must be to monitor inequalities amongst older people, as is already done with mortality rates by social class for people of working age. This monitoring was seen as crucial by Acheson's committee that reviewed health inequalities in Britain in the early 1990s [67]. However, in so doing, it needs to be remembered that reporting of self-rated health and of functioning may be affected by cultural expectations and values as well as by objective illnesses, impairment, and individual personality. This could influence apparent trends but different theories predict different divergences. First, people in advantaged situations may be more likely to rate themselves in poor health because they have higher ideals, have greater affinity with the medical profession, and expect treatment [68,69]. If this is true, interventions to encourage health promotion amongst the disadvantaged groups could initially widen the observed gap as they learn to state their health problems more fully. On the other hand, disadvantaged people may be more reliant on physical functioning to get by in daily life and so have greater motivation to report difficulties [68]. If this is true, then even with a major improvement in the functioning of the more disadvantaged people, a measured difference in self-reported quality of life or self-rated health will remain.

Monitoring is insufficient. There are several stages of the progress of health inequalities at which intervention can be targeted. Link and Phelan [70] argue that, historically, the diseases and risk factors that dominate health inequalities have changed, but each time people with monetary and educational resources are the first to reduce their risk factor profile. Therefore, it could be more effective in the long run to reduce differences in income and education than to focus on proximal risk factors. However, comparisons between the United Kingdom and both Sweden and Finland show that having a good welfare system or employment support and redistributive income policies do not suffice to remove differences in health between groups who are disadvantaged in other respects (occupation or being a lone mother) [71,72]. Material resources alone are unlikely to suffice without adequate coping mechanisms, including the will to continue, and belief in self-efficacy.

Meanwhile, it would be neglectful of the current older generations not to try to reduce inequalities. Part of this should be encouragement of healthier lifestyles. Unfortunately, this is not straightforward. For example, Ebrahim and Davey Smith [73] pointed out that interventions aimed at improving individual risk profiles for cardiovascular disease have been limited in effect and costly. Apparently 'unhealthy' behaviour may be justifiable for some older people (e.g., cannot afford health food or find it difficult to eat) and health education does not necessarily change this. There have to be broader changes that make the behaviour appropriate for them. Another policy goal should be to improve health and social services that can bring major benefits to those already experiencing some impairment or disability [74].

There is much we do not yet know about the effectiveness and potential impact of interventions, particularly community interventions. For example, few studies have looked into health impact of housing interventions for people of any age [75,76] or dietary interventions for the elderly [77].

Sustained effort is needed to make a lasting impact on health differentials in older age, and a long-term view is required that is not overly influenced by the exigencies of short-term political agendas.

References

1. Sutherland, S., With respect to old age: Long term care—Rights and responsibilities, Report of The Royal Commission on Long Term Care, Cm 4192-I, 1-196, Norwich, The Stationery Office, 1999.
2. Department of Health, National Service Framework for Older People, London, Department of Health, National Service Frameworks, 2001.
3. Kunst, A.E. and Mackenbach, J.P., Measuring socioeconomic inequalities in health, World Health Organisation, Copenhagen, 1995.
4. Woodward, A. and Kawachi, I., Why reduce health inequalities? *J Epidemiol Community Health*, 54, 923, 2000.
5. Vaillant, G.E. and Mukamal, K., Successful aging, *Am J Psychiatry*, 158, 839, 2001.
6. Kaplan, G.A., Maintenance of functioning in the elderly, *Ann Epidemiol*, 2, 823, 1992.
7. Rogers, R.G., Rogers, A., and Belanger, A., Disability-free life among the elderly in the United States, *J Aging Health*, 4, 19, 1992.
8. Maddox, G.L., Clark, D.O., and Steinhauser, K., Dynamics of functional impairment in late adulthood, *Soc Sci Med*, 38, 925, 1994.
9. Crimmins, E.M. and Saito, Y., Getting better and getting worse. Transitions in functional status among older Americans, *J Aging Health*, 5, 3, 1993.
10. Beckett, L.A., Brock, D.B., Lemke, J.H., Mendes de Leon, C.F., Guralnik, J.M., Fillenbaum, G.G., Branch, L.G., Wetle, T.T., and Evans, D.A., Analysis of change in self-reported physical function among older persons in four population studies, *Am J Epidemiol*, 143, 766, 1996.
11. Black, D., Morris, J.N., Smith, C., and Townsend, P., *Inequalities in health: The Black Report*, London, Penguin Books, 1992, 31.
12. Macintyre, S., The patterning of health by social position in contemporary Britain: Directions for sociological research, *Soc Sci Med*, 23, 393, 1986.
13. Fox, A.J., Goldblatt, P.O., and Adelstein, A.M., Selection and mortality differentials, *J Epidemiol Community Health*, 36, 69, 1982.
14. Bartley, M. and Plewis, I., Does health-selective mobility account for socioeconomic differences in health? Evidence from England and Wales, 1971 to 1991, *J Health Soc Behav*, 38, 376, 1997.
15. Blane, D., Harding, S., and Rosato, M., Does social mobility affect the size of the mortality differential? Evidence from the Office for National Statistics Longitudinal Study, *J R Stat Soc A*, 162, 59, 1999.
16. Davey Smith, G., Blane, D., and Bartley, M., Explanations for socioeconomic differentials in mortality, *Eur J Public Health*, 4, 131, 1994.
17. Nillsson, P.M., Møller, L., and Östergen, P.-O., Social class and cardiovascular disease—An update, *Scand J Soc Med*, 23, 3, 1995.
18. Elstad, J.I., The psychosocial perspective on social inequalities in health. In: *The sociology of health inequalities*, ed. Bartley, M., Blane, D., and Davey Smith, D. Oxford, Blackwell Publishers Ltd, 1998, 35.

19. Brunner, E., Towards a new social biology. In: *Social epidemiology*, ed. Berkman, L.F. and Kawachi, I. Oxford, Oxford University Press, 2000, 306.
20. Wilkinson, R.G., *Unhealthy societies. The afflictions of inequality*, London, Routledge, 1996.
21. Kuh, D. and Ben-Shlomo, Y., Introduction: A lifecourse approach to the aetiology of chronic disease. In: *A lifecourse approach to the chronic disease epidemiology*, ed. Kuh, D. and Ben-Shlomo, Y. Oxford, Oxford University Press, 1997, 6.
22. Davey Smith, G., Socioeconomic differentials. In: *A lifecourse approach to the chronic disease epidemiology*, ed. Kuh, D. and Ben-Shlomo, Y. Oxford, Oxford University Press, 1997, 242.
23. Galobardes, B. et al., Indicators of socioeconomic position (part 1), *J Epidemiol Community Health*, 60, 7, 2006.
24. Galobardes, B. et al., Indicators of socioeconomic position (part 2), *J Epidemiol Community Health*, 60, 95, 2006.
25. Breeze, E., Sloggett, A., and Fletcher, A., Socioeconomic and demographic predictors of mortality and institutional residence among middle aged and older people: Results from the Longitudinal Study, *J Epidemiol Community Health*, 53, 765, 1999.
26. Breeze, E., Sloggett, A., and Fletcher, A., Socioeconomic status and transitions in status in old age in relation to limiting long-term illness measured at the 1991 Census: Results from the U.K. Longitudinal Study, *Eur J Public Health*, 9, 265, 1999.
27. Clarke, R. et al., Design, objectives, and lessons from a pilot 25-year follow-up resurvey of survivors in the Whitehall Study of London Civil Servants, *J Epidemiol Community Health*, 52, 364, 1998.
28. Breeze, E. et al., Do socioeconomic disadvantages persist into old age? Self-reported morbidity in a 29-year follow-up of the Whitehall Study, *Am J Public Health*, 91, 277, 2001.
29. Bergner, M., Bobbitt, R.A., Carter, W.B., and Gilson, B.S., The Sickness Impact Profile: Development and final revision of a health status measure, *Med Care*, XIX, 787, 1981.
30. Lawton, M.P., The Philadelphia Geriatric Center Morale Scale: A revision, *J Gerontol*, 30, 85, 1975.
31. Breeze, E. et al., Association of quality of life in old age in Britain with socioeconomic position: Baseline data from a randomised controlled trial. *J Epidemiol Community Health*, 58, 667, 2004.
32. Fletcher, A., Jones, D., Bulpitt, C., and Tulloch, A., The MRC trial of assessment and management of older people in the community: Objectives, design and interventions, *BMC Health Serv Res*, 2, 21, 2002.
33. Marmot, M.G. and Shipley, M.J., Do socioeconomic differences in mortality persist after retirement? 25-year follow up of civil servants from the first Whitehall Study, *Br Med J*, 313, 1177, 1996.
34. Moore, D.E. and Hayward, M.D., Occupational careers and mortality of elderly men, *Demography*, 27, 31, 1990.
35. Olausson, P.O., Mortality among the elderly in Sweden by social class, *Soc Sci Med*, 32, 437, 1991.
36. Guralnik, J.M. and Kaplan, G.A., Predictors of healthy aging: Prospective evidence from the Alameda County study, *Am J Public Health*, 79, 703, 1989.

37. Camacho,T. et al., Functional ability in the oldest old. Cumulative impact of risk factors from the previous two decades, *J Aging Health*, 5, 439, 1993.

38. Reed, D.M. et al., Predictors of healthy aging in men with high life expectancies, *Am J Public Health*, 88, 1463, 1998.

39. Keil, J.E. et al., Predictors of physical disability in elderly blacks and whites of the Charleston Heart Study, *J Clin Epidemiol*, 42, 521, 1989.

40. Parker, M.G., Thorslund, M., and Lundberg, O., Physical function and social class among Swedish oldest old, *J Gerontol*, 49, S196, 1994.

41. Parker, M.G. et al., Predictors of physical function among the oldest old: A comparison of three outcome variables in a 24-year follow-up, *J Aging Health*, 8, 444, 1996.

42. Thorslund, M. and Lundberg, O., Health and inequalities among the oldest old, *J Aging Health*, 6, 51, 1994.

43. Victor, C.R., Inequalities in health in later life, *Age Ageing*, 18, 387, 1989.

44. Blaxter, M., *Health and lifestyles*, London, Tavistock/Routledge, 1990, 66.

45. Arber, S. and Ginn, J., Gender and inequalities in health in later life, *Soc Sci Med*, 36, 33, 1993.

46. Falaschetti, E., Malbut, K., and Primatesta, P., *The general health of older people and their use of health services*, Norwich, The Stationery Office, 2002.

47. Hirani, V. and Malbut, K., *Disability among older people*, Norwich, The Stationery Office, 2002.

48. Berkman, C.S. and Gurland, B.J., The relationship among income, other socioeconomic indicators, and functional level in older persons, *J Aging Health*, 10, 81, 1998.

49. Dahl, E. and Birkelund, G.E., Health inequalities in later life in a social democratic welfare state, *Soc Sci Med*, 44, 871, 1997.

50. Damian, J. et al., Determinants of self assessed health among Spanish older people living at home, *J Epidemiol Community Health*, 53, 412, 1999.

51. Sakari-Rantala, R., Heikkinen, E., and Ruoppila, I., Difficulties in mobility among elderly people and their association with socioeconomic factors, dwelling environment and use of services, *Aging* (Milano), 7, 433, 1995.

52. Goldblatt, P., Mortality and alternative social classifications. In 1971–1981 Longitudinal Study. Mortality and Social Organisation, 1990, 192.

53. Filakti, H. and Fox, J., Differences in mortality by housing tenure and by car access from the OPCS Longitudinal Study, *Popul Trends*, 27, 1995.

54. Smith, J. and Harding, S., Mortality of women and men using alternative social classifications. In: *Health inequalities*, ed. Drever, F. and Whitehead, M. London, The Stationery Office, 1997, 168.

55. Salas, C., On the empirical association between poor health and low socioeconomic status at old age, *Health Econ*, 11, 207, 2002.

56. Rogot, E., Sorlie, P.D., and Johnson, N.J., Life expectancy by employment status, income, and education, the National Longitudinal Mortality Study Public Health Rep, 107, 457, 1992.

57. Manor, O., Eisenbach, Z., Peritz, E., and Friedlander, Y., Mortality differentials among Israeli men, *Am J Public Health*, 89, 1807, 1999.

58. Martikainen, P. et al., Income differences in mortality: a register-based follow-up study of three million men and women, *Int J Epidemiol*, 30, 1397, 2001.

59. Van Rossum, C.T.M. et al., Socioeconomic status and mortality in Dutch elderly people, *Eur J Public Health*, 10, 255, 2000.

60. Swain, V.J., Changes in self-reported health. In: *The Health and Lifestyle Survey: Seven years on*, ed. Cox, B.D., Huppert, F.A., and Whichelow, M.J. Dartmouth, Aldershot, 1993, 49.

61. Harris, T. et al., Longitudinal study of physical ability in the oldest-old, *Am J Public Health*, 79, 698, 1989.

62. Strawbridge, W.J., Cohen, R.D., Shema, S.J., and Kaplan, G.A., Successful aging: Predictors and associated activities, *Am J Epidemiol*, 144, 135, 1996.

63. Maddox, G.L. and Clark, D.O., Trajectories of functional impairment in later life, *J Health Soc Behav*, 33, 114, 1992.

64. Melzer, D. et al., Educational differences in the prevalence of mobility disability in old age: The dynamics of incidence, mortality, and recovery, *J Gerontol B Psychol Sci Soc Sci*, 56, S294, 2001.

65. Roos, N.P. and Havens, B., Predictors of successful aging: A twelve-year study of Manitoba elderly, *Am J Public Health*, 81, 63, 1991.

66. Palmore, E.B., Nowlin, J.B., and Wang, H.S., Predictors of function among the old-old: A 10-year follow-up, *J Gerontol*, 40, 244, 1985.

67. Acheson, D. et al., *Independent inquiry into inequalities in health*. London, The Stationery Office, 1998, 30.

68. Elstad, J.I., How large are the differences—really? Self-reported long-standing illness among working class and middle class men, *Sociol Health Illness*, 18, 475, 1996.

69. Blane, D., Power, C., and Bartley, M., The measurement of morbidity in relation to social class. In: *Medical sociology: Research on chronic illness*, ed. Abel, T. Bonn/Berlin, Informationszentrum Sozialwissenschaften, 1993, 65.

70. Link, B.G. and Phelan, J., Social conditions as fundamental causes of disease. *J Health Soc Behav*, Spec No, 80, 1995.

71. Whitehead, M., Burstrom, B., and Diderichsen, F., Social policies and the pathways to inequalities in health: A comparative analysis of lone mothers in Britain and Sweden, *Soc Sci Med*, 50, 255, 2000.

72. Martikainen, P. and Valkonen, T., Inequalities in health. Policies to reduce income inequalities are unlikely to eradicate inequalities in mortality, *Br Med J (Clin Res Ed)*, 319, 319, 1999.

73. Ebrahim, S. and Smith, G.D., Systematic review of randomised controlled trials of multiple risk factor interventions for preventing coronary heart disease, *Br Med J*, 14, 1666, 1997.

74. Fletcher, A., Breeze, E., and Walters, R., Political challenges 1. The ageing issue: Health promotion for elderly people. In: *The evidence of health promotion effectiveness. Shaping public health in Europe*, ed. Black, D. Paris, IUHPE, 1999, 12.

75. Thomson, H., Petticrew, M., and Morrison, D., Health effects of housing improvement: Systematic review of intervention studies, *Br Med J*, 323, 187, 2001.

76. Taske N. et al., Housing and public health: A review of reviews of interventions for improving health, London, National Institute for Health and Clinical Excellence. Evidence briefing, 2005, 1.

77. Fletcher, A. and Rake, C. Effectiveness of interventions to promote healthy eating in the elderly. People living in the community, London, Health Education Authority, 1998.

chapter eight

Demographic change, family support, and ageing well: developed country perspectives

Emily M.D. Grundy

Contents

Introduction 85
Population ageing and kin networks 86
    Demographic change and kin networks 87
Family support 91
    Living arrangements and intergenerational co-residence...................91
    Contacts and provision of support 93
Consequences of family support..96
    Family support and health...96
    Family support and use of services..97
Looking to the future 98
References..99

Introduction

In several countries in Europe, the world region with the oldest population, a quarter of the population will be aged sixty-five years or over by 2020. In many, numbers and proportions of very old people are growing particularly rapidly, and United Nations projections suggest that by 2050 there will be nineteen countries, including Britain, France, Germany, Italy, Japan, and Spain, in which at least 10% of the population is aged eighty or more [1].

The assumption of policy makers is that these demographic changes will mean that younger people will need to make larger contributions of various kinds to provide for the old. These contributions will include not just higher taxes to pay for pensions and health care, but also more family care and support [2]. Most people aged sixty-five and over do not have disabling health problems but, in later old age, rates of morbidity, disability, and needs for assistance are high; for example, a quarter of women aged eighty-five and over in Britain are unable to bathe or shower without assistance and half are unable to manage one or more locomotion activities without help [3]. There are indications of declines in disability at older ages in at least some countries and also improvements in the environment (such as in housing and heating) that have diminished needs for help with some tasks [4,5]. However, even projections that assume falling rates of disability show large increases in the number of dependent older people (with limitations in activities of daily living [ADLs]—tasks such as bathing, dressing, and transferring to and from bed) as a result of growth in the size of the age groups in which the prevalence of disability is greatest [6].

Currently, most of the help needed by older people with disabilities is provided by family members (including elderly family members such as spouses) even in countries with well developed health and social care systems [5,7–10]. However, interrelated with the demographic shifts partly driving age structure changes have been substantial changes in family and household patterns. These have been perceived as a symptom of and a contributor to weakening family bonds, with potential negative effects on the family support of older people [11]; in short, there are concerns that the availability of family care for older people may decline just as the numbers needing it increase. Such a change would have implications for older people's needs for services and for their well-being more generally because family ties form a major element of many older people's social environment. Extensive and growing evidence indicates that this social environment, including social participation and social support, is an important component of ageing well [12].

In this chapter this issue is examined from several perspectives. First, the underlying demographic trends and their effects on population age structure and on the proportion of older people with close relatives, notably spouses and children, are presented. Second, the current patterns of family support are considered. Finally, the linkages between family household, and social support, and health and well-being in later life are discussed and implications for the future are examined.

Population ageing and kin networks

In Britain and a number of other Northern and Western European countries, the transition from relatively high to low fertility set in motion towards the end of the nineteenth century produced a shift to an older structure in the first half of the twentieth century. In England and Wales, for example, the proportion of the population aged sixty-five and over doubled from 5 to 10% in the first half of the twentieth century. Fertility fell later—but faster and further—in Southern and Eastern European countries, although many of these shared the postwar baby boom of the late 1950s and early 1960s [13]. Several European countries and Japan now have total fertility rates (an indicator of how many children a woman would have at current rates) well below 1.5 (and below the level for England and Wales, which in 2005 was 1.8). These trends, if continued, will lead to further population ageing and natural decrease in population size.

Improvements in mortality rates are also contributing to accelerated population ageing. In developed countries most deaths occur at older ages and reductions in the overall level of mortality are being achieved through improved survival beyond the age of sixty-five. These improvements have been considerable (except in Eastern Europe) and in several countries have recently been greater for men than for women, a reversal of a long previous trend towards increasing female advantage in mortality. In England and Wales, for example, male life expectancy at age sixty-five increased by less than two years between 1901 and 1971 (from 10.1 to 11.9 years) but then by over four years between 1971 and 2001 (to 16). For women, gains were more evenly spread over the century with an increase of nearly six years between 1901 and 1971 (from 11.1 to 15.8) and a further gain of just over three years (to 19.1) over the next three decades [3].

Demographic change and kin networks

The demographic changes that have led to population ageing have also resulted in changes in the structure and size of kin networks [14]. In terms of availability of spouses and children—the most important potential supporters of older people—prospects for the next twenty to thirty years in Britain and many other European countries are in fact favourable. Marriage rates and proportions, especially of women, of those who never married were much higher amongst cohorts born in the late nineteenth and early twentieth centuries than in the later born cohorts, with those born in the 1930s and 1940s leading something of a marriage boom [13,15,16].

As a result, as shown in Table 8.1, the proportions of married women in England and Wales have been increasing and are projected to increase further, whilst the proportions of those never married are reducing. For example, in 1971, 16% of women aged eighty-five and over were never married, compared with 10% in 2001 and a projected low of 6% in 2021. Moreover, falling late age mortality and particularly the big falls in mortality of older men seen in England and Wales and several other countries have served to postpone widowhood. These changes are less pronounced amongst men (amongst whom the proportion of never married is projected to increase slightly), but, overall, in the next twenty years the numbers of married older people will increase faster than the older population as a whole.

Table 8.1 Distribution (%) of Population Aged Seventy-Five and Over by Marital Status, 1971–2031, England and Wales

	Men				Women			
	Single	Married	Widowed	Divorced	Single	Married	Widowed	Divorced
1971	6	58	35	—	15	19	65	—
1991	7	63	28	—	11	23	64	—
2001	7	63	27	3	7	25	64	3
2021	6	62	22	10	4	33	52	11
2031	9	60	19	12	6	37	43	15

Source: ONS population estimates and GAD 2003-based population projections by legal marital status.

Partly as a consequence of these trends in marriage, levels of fertility were also higher and levels of childlessness lower amongst women born in the 1930s and 1940s than in earlier (or later) cohorts. This may seem surprising, given the role of falling fertility in driving population ageing, but as already noted, in Britain and a number of other European countries, the initial shift to lower fertility occurred in the late nineteenth or early twentieth century. Although fertility levels have never returned to pretransition levels, there have since then been periods of higher fertility (for example, during the postwar baby boom). The distribution of family sizes has also changed. In England and Wales, the *average* number of children produced by women born in 1900 and women born in 1955 was the same —two—but the earlier cohort included a higher proportion of women with four or more children and also a higher proportion with no or only one child [13,16].

The cohorts born in the 1930s and 1940s—the parents of the baby boom—had higher fertility than those born earlier or later in the twentieth century and lower proportions childless. This is shown in Figure 8.1, for England and Wales, and presents the parity distribution of women born between 1920 and 1960. A fifth of the 1920 cohort had no children (and amongst cohorts born at the beginning of the twentieth century this proportion was even higher) compared with half as many amongst those born in 1945. Moreover, as a result of lower levels of mortality, more of these children have survived or will survive to their mother's later old age.

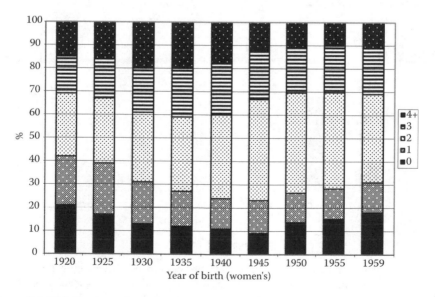

Figure 8.1 Distribution of women by year of birth and parity at age forty-five, England and Wales. (From National Statistics.)

Results from demographic modelling show that in England and Wales some 90% of women born in 1946 will have at least one child still alive when they reach the age of eighty (in 2026), compared with less than 82% amongst those born in 1926 who constitute today's population of eighty-year-olds; indeed, the proportion of older women with at least one living child available is likely to be higher in the next quarter century than in any earlier (or, most probably, any later) period [17]. Similar patterns have been demonstrated for a number of other European countries [18]. This trend will reverse when the cohorts born from the mid-1950s onwards reach older age.

Falling mortality has also led to the longer co-survival of parents and adult children and contributed to the 'verticalisation' of family structures. A national survey conducted in Britain in 1999 found three quarters of all adults were members of families including at least three living generations and that, as shown in Figure 8.2, a third of people aged eighty and over had at least one child, one grandchild, and one great-grandchild alive [19]. Recent modelling work suggests that in Britain the proportion of women aged sixty with a mother still alive will continue to increase until the cohort born in the 1970s reach this age [17]. In the longer term, however, continuing declines in late age mortality will be offset by recent trends to delay fertility and consequent longer gaps between generations, which will slow down or even reverse the trend towards verticalisation.

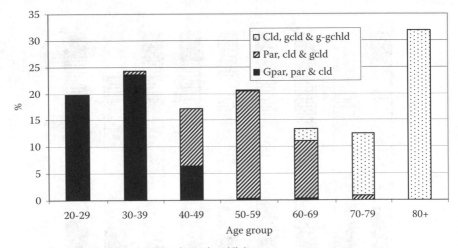

Source: Omnibus Survey data in Grundy, Murphy and Shelton

Figure 8.2 Proportion (%) of adults in families including three living generations, Britain 1999. (From Omnibus Survey data in Grundy, E. et al., *Population Trends*, 97, 19, 1999.)

Different sections of the population have differing patterns of fertility and mortality, so there are considerable variations within countries (as well as between them) in kin networks. In general, higher status groups have lower mortality and later (and lower) fertility. The 1999 British survey of kin and kin contacts referred to earlier found that 45% of forty-five- to sixty-nine-year-olds from white-collar groups had a living parent compared with only 23% of blue-collar respondents; similar results have been reported from the United States and elsewhere [20].

These demographic trends mean that in the next twenty to thirty years the potential family support available to older people will tend to increase. It is important to note too that older people are important providers of support, and, indeed, within families the balance of transfers tends to flow downward from older generations at least until the age of seventy or seventy-five [21,22]. These downward transfers include money and provision of practical help, including help with grandchildren. The greater availability of older generation relatives thus brings benefits as well as potential costs for their children and grandchildren. Longer term prospects for the demographic availability of close kin are, however, much less favourable because cohorts born since the mid-1950s have experienced high rates of divorce, as well as a return to higher levels of childlessness and lower nuptiality.

Demographic availability of close kin is a necessary, but not always a sufficient, requirement for the provision of family support and many questions have been raised about possible changes in the willingness or ability of younger generations to provide assistance. These concerns have been partly fuelled by major changes in the living arrangements of older people, especially unmarried older people.

Family support

Living arrangements and intergenerational co-residence

In the 1950s and 1960s it was quite common for older widowed people to live with a child, even in Scandinavia, other Northwest European countries, and North America [8,23]. Now, even in very old age groups, living alone is the most usual arrangement for women without a spouse. In England and Wales in 2001, for example, 55% of women aged eighty-five and over lived alone, 9% lived with a spouse, and only 13% lived with other relatives—considerably fewer than the 23% living in some kind of institutional care [24]. Men have the substantial advantage of being far more likely to be married even in later old age and the proportions in this age group living alone or in an institution were much lower—32 and 13%, respectively—but the former is still high in a historical context.

The extent of the decline in intergenerational co-residence is illustrated in Figure 8.3, which shows for 1971 and 2001 the proportion of the older private household (noninstitutional) population that lived in households containing at least two generations. Changes have been particularly marked

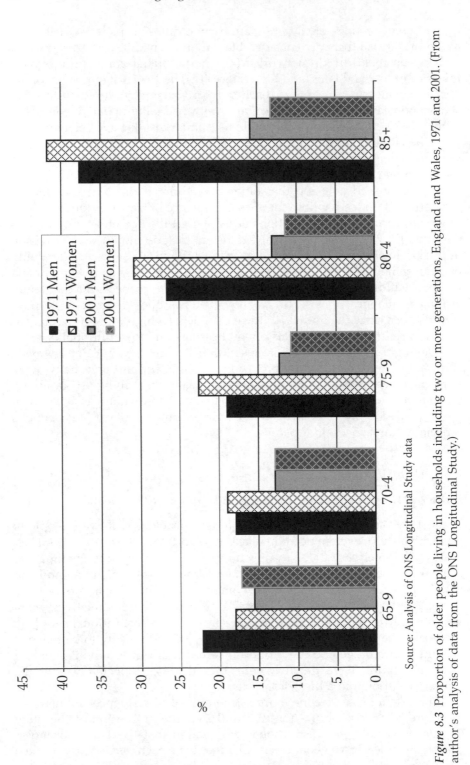

Source: Analysis of ONS Longitudinal Study data

Figure 8.3 Proportion of older people living in households including two or more generations, England and Wales, 1971 and 2001. (From author's analysis of data from the ONS Longitudinal Study.)

amongst the older old: Thus, the proportion of women aged eighty-five and over who lived in a multigenerational household fell from 42% in 1971 to 13% in 2001. Trends in other industrialised countries are similar, although the extent of co-residence continues to vary and is generally higher in Southern Europe (and Austria and Ireland) and in Japan than in Northwest Europe or North America, and lowest of all in the Nordic countries [24–28]. As co-residence with relatives has declined, the proportions of people living alone or just with a spouse have increased.

At one time, declines in the availability of kin with whom to co-reside were thought to partly account for the trend towards residential independence amongst older people. However, as discussed previously, the availability of a spouse and at least one child has tended to increase rather than diminish since the 1970s (although declines in the proportion of older people with large families will have led to some reduction in the proportions with a child with the characteristics most associated with intergenerational co-residence).

Rather than being demographically driven, the increased residential independence of the older population is now generally attributed to an increasing number of older people now being able to afford to maintain a separate home and to increasing preferences for separate living; improvements in health may also have had some influence. The sizeable variations between countries and between groups of differing heritages within countries points to the continuing importance of cultural factors [25–28]. For example, intergenerational co-residence is much more usual in Southern than in Northern Europe and this differential is evident even when number of children is taken into account [28,29]. Ethnicity, religion, and ancestry are also associated with within-country differences in living arrangements in North America and in Europe [30,31].

Contacts and provision of support

Although intergenerational co-residence has plummeted, extensive survey evidence points to high levels of contact and mutual support between older people and their families, even if living separately [5,8,10,21,22,32–34]. Frequent contact is more common in Southern than Northern European countries. Results from the recent Survey of Health and Retirement in Europe (SHARE) conducted in ten European countries in 2004, for example, showed that, in the Southern European countries surveyed, at least three quarters of parents aged eighty and over were in touch with a child daily. This proportion was much lower in the Netherlands, Sweden, and Denmark, but was still at least 20–40% (being lower amongst men) [34].

The 2002 English Longitudinal Survey of Ageing, with a similar design to SHARE, reported that 63% of mothers and 55% of fathers aged seventy-five and over met up with children at least weekly [35]. Information on trends in contact is sparse, but comparisons of the proportion of adult children seeing a parent at least weekly found in the 1999 British survey of kin and kin contacts with results from similar surveys undertaken in 1986 and 1994 showed no evidence of a trend towards reduced contact [36]. Older people and their relatives are also involved in frequent exchanges of help, often reciprocal, with tasks and activities such as shopping, paperwork, household chores, and, in the case of help provided by older people, care of grandchildren [21,22,37].

Within countries, those from more highly educated groups tend to have less contact with relatives and also different patterns of support exchanges, and help from younger to older generations is more pronounced in less advantaged groups [22,37]. However, the association between socioeconomic status and family exchange seems to be less pronounced in Southern than in Northern Europe [27,33]. Gender, marital status, and, in the case of children's contacts with parents, number of siblings and parental marital status are all also associated with levels of contact and exchanges of help.

This is illustrated for Britain in Table 8.2, which shows results from analyses of variations in the proportion of adult children with at least weekly face-to-face contact with mothers and fathers (of those with a mother or father alive). Proximity is, as would be expected, a strong influence, but how close a parent and child live to each other may be a consequence, rather than a cause, of desired interaction patterns. For this reason, the table shows the results of models including and excluding this variable. Contact and provision of help were positively associated with lower socioeconomic status (of the adult child) and with the child being a daughter, and negatively associated with the child's age and with the number of siblings (a finding suggesting people adjust their contacts with parents taking account of parents' contacts with other children). Daughters had more contact with mothers than with fathers and were less likely to see their father frequently if their mother was dead. Paternal divorce was also strongly associated with less contact and support. Similar findings have been reported from a range of studies in other European and North American countries [21,37,38].

Apart from help with everyday tasks and sharing of activities, some midlife children provide more extensive care for disabled older parents. Ogg and Renault [39] found that between 6 and 13% of people aged fifty to fifty-nine included in the SHARE surveys who had a parent alive were providing personal care.

It seems from the evidence reviewed earlier that in the short-term future, relatively more of the older population of Britain and many other countries will have the potential support of a spouse or child to draw on than has been the case in the past (or will be the case in the longer term future); although intergenerational co-residence has become much less usual, levels of contact and mutual help between older parents and their children (and grandchildren) are high, although with variations between and within countries. In the final sections of this chapter, the implications of these conclusions are considered in terms of influences on older people's health, well-being, and access to care when it is needed.

Table 8.2 Odds Ratios from Logistic Regression Analysis of Variations in the Proportion of Adult Children Aged Twenty-Five to Fifty-Four Giving Regular Help to Parents

	Excluding proximity		Including proximity	
	Provides help to mother	Provides help to father	Provides help to mother	Provides help to father
(Intercept)	1.320	0.458[a]	0.914	0.366[b]
Respondent female (ref. male)	0.929	1.470[c]	0.920	1.580[a]
Education:				
High (ref.)	1.000	1.000	—	—
Medium	1.520[b]	1.480[a]	—	—
Low	1.230	1.750[a]	—	—
Parental marital history:				
First marriage (ref.)	1.000	1.000	1.000	1.000
2+ marriage	0.827	0.453[b]	0.826	0.530[b]
Divorced/ separated/never married	1.370	0.541[a]	1.810[a]	0.693
Widowed	1.550[b]	1.390	1.570[b]	1.590[c]
Lives in North (ref. South)	—	1.300[a]	0.819	—
Siblings:				
None (ref.)	—	1.000	1.000	1.000
One	—	0.778	—	0.830
Two or more	—	0.998	—	1.140
Social class (ref. I and II):				
I and II (ref.)	1.000	1.000	1.000	1.000
IIIN-M	1.200	0.871	0.966	0.745
IIIM	1.120	1.160	0.882	1.050
IV,V	0.968	0.897	0.789	0.788
Unclassified	0.303[b]	0.238[a]	0.266[b]	0.262[a]
Lives near parent	—	—	5.160[b]	3.840[b]
N	1,430	1,080	1,430	1,080

Notes: Long dash (—) indicates variable not significant and so not included in final model. Model controls for respondents' and parents' ages. Excludes children co-resident with parents.

[a] Significant at 5% level.

[b] Significant at 1% level.

[c] Significant at 10% level.

Consequences of family support

Family support and health

A large body of research points to links between social engagement and support, measured and conceptualised in a variety of ways, and a range of health and well-being outcomes. Although there are some inconsistencies in the literature, researchers have reported associations between indicators of social linkages and outcomes including mortality, physical and psychological morbidity, cognitive function, recovery from acute illness, and use of health services and medication (see, for example, reviews by Bowling and Grundy [40] and Bath and Deeg [12]). Studies have found links between both perceived emotional support and engagement in wider social networks and social activities (including those not involving enhancement of physical fitness) and indicators of health [41–47].

Given the important role of family members as confidantes, helpers, and members of social networks, it would seem an obvious conclusion that family support and engagement should also contribute positively to the health and well-being of older people. Evidence for this is strongest in the case of availability of a spouse. Numerous studies have indicated that marriage seems to be associated with clear health benefits for older men, with married men generally having the best health and lowest mortality (for reviews, see McIntyre [48] and Waite [49]). Results for older women are less clear-cut; some studies have found no advantage for the married or, indeed, advantages for the never married women [43,50]. This may be because women have stronger links with friends and other relatives and so are less reliant on spouses for emotional support; never married women in particular may be able to draw on alternative social networks cultivated over a lifetime [51].

Information on the effects of relationships with children and other relatives on health and well-being is surprisingly sparse and also harder to interpret, due to the complexity of various selective influences. Analysis of data from the Berlin Ageing Study, for example, showed that keeping in touch with relatives was associated with better social functioning and less risk of loneliness but, as pointed out by the author, this could be because more socially outgoing and emotionally stable individuals are more likely to maintain these linkages [52].

A recent study from the United States suggested that, amongst lower educated men, the perceived availability of support from a child was associated with better scores on a health index; the effect was such that men of low education who had such support had health as good as more highly educated men [45]. Similar effects were not found for women; this seems surprising given the gendered nature of close kin relationships but may reflect women's larger alternative networks of supportive friends. Results from the longitudinal Copenhagen City Heart Study showed that parents with less than monthly contact with children had higher mortality and a higher incidence of ischaemic heart disease; again, these effects were stronger for men than women. Availability of a spouse or partner was also associated with better outcomes [53].

However, a recent cross-sectional analysis of data from the English Longitudinal Study of Ageing suggested that greater contacts with children and other relatives had a negative effect on quality of life [54]. This may be because children and other supporters tend to increase contacts with older relatives experiencing health and other difficulties, may reflect the effect of worrying about children and grandchildren, or may be because the quality of life scale used in this study (which included four dimensions representing control, autonomy, self-realisation, and pleasure) may be biased towards individualistic rather than familial components of quality of life. Although participation in social activities appears to be associated with preservation of cognitive function (and such activities may be undertaken with a child), a recent carefully controlled longitudinal study of Taiwanese elderly people found no association between numbers of close relatives contacted at least weekly and later cognitive performance [47].

Family support and use of services

Married people potentially have access to practical help and care from a spouse, as well as emotional support, and children are also potential care providers for older people with disabilities. The proportion of married older people in or entering institutional care is much lower than that of older people of other marital statuses, particularly the never married (who in current older cohorts are generally childless) [55,56]. Availability of a child—particularly a daughter—is associated with differentials in use of institutional care and other formal services [7,56]. Living with a spouse or other co-resident (usually an adult child), especially a spouse in good health, is also associated with a greater chance of dying at home—a preferred option amongst older individuals [57].

Availability of children is, of course, also a prerequisite of co-residence with a child. Whether or not this is regarded as a desirable (or least undesirable) option for older people with serious disabilities and major assistance needs will depend on a range of personal and cultural preferences and circumstances and the availability and quality of alternatives, such as nursing home care. In Southern European countries, older people who live with their adult children report higher levels of satisfaction than other women [27], whereas a study conducted in Wales found that older people living with relatives were the most likely to report loneliness and poor morale [51]. This may reflect cultural differences in preferences and different pathways to co-residence; in countries, such as Britain, where residential independence is valued, co-residence with a child may more often be a last resort than a positive choice.

Different pathways to specific types of living arrangements also make it difficult to unravel possible effects on health. Most studies (for a review, see Grundy [58]) that have looked at this find that in older groups those living with a spouse have the best health, consistent with the literature on marital status differences in health, and that, especially amongst the older old, those living alone are in better health than those living with relatives. However, this is presumably because serious disability makes living alone very difficult and is an important driver of changes in living arrangements. Some recent longitudinal studies conducted in Scandinavia and the United States that have controlled carefully for initial health status have found some indications of health-damaging effects of living alone (the usual option for the unmarried in Northern European and American populations), including cognitive decline, especially in groups with serious impairments at baseline [42,59]. Higher risks of cognitive decline have also been reported amongst those with no close social ties, those with unsatisfactory relationships with close relatives, and those with few social activities [42,47].

From a policy perspective, a crucial question is whether providing more formal support services 'crowds out' family care or, conversely, whether the provision of support to family carers enables more care for a longer period. In general, most analysts who have examined this issue have concluded that providing more services to older people at home does not displace family support, although it may lead to some changes in focus [60,61]. In Scotland, for example, the recent introduction of free personal care seems to have resulted in some family supporters switching from providing personal care to spending more time on other types of support, such as help with shopping and domestic chores [62].

In many European countries with developed welfare states, care shared by family and formal providers appears most usual (and generally pre-ferred), although the balance between the two varies and clearly may change in response to expansion or contraction in availability of the other element. In some countries, for example, recent targeting of home care services on the most seriously disabled older people (and consequent reduction in ser-vices for those with lesser disabilities) has led to families of the latter having to increase their efforts [5]. Countries such as Denmark with a relatively high provision of home care services also have higher than average proportions of older disabled people with a professional rather than a family carer and high—and increasing—expressed preferences for professional rather than family help with personal care [9,32].

Looking to the future

Older people rate relationships with family members high amongst the domains of life important to them and the available empirical evidence shows that most people are in close contact with family members and engaged in various, generally reciprocal, exchanges of support. Emotional support and social engagement are known to be important dimensions of a healthy old age and it seems highly probable that family links form a major component of these, although empirical evidence on this (apart from evidence on the role of marriage) is surprisingly sparse. Family support is, of course, particularly important for older people with disabilities who need assistance, and there is evidence that availability of such support influences uses of services such as institutional care, although providing help for older people does not necessarily displace family help.

Increases in the proportion of older people with a spouse and at least one child, projected for the next twenty to thirty years, are therefore positive developments for older people and society as a whole. The demographic context in the longer term future, when the post-1950 cohorts reach later life is less favourable because these cohorts will have experienced more diverse partnership histories and a return to higher levels of childlessness. Whether or not stronger friendship networks will be able to compensate for fewer family ties, as sometimes suggested, is as yet unclear. These trends suggest an urgent need during the relatively auspicious next couple of decades to research and establish the best means of enabling older people to maintain and develop supportive relationships and social activities, the best balance between formal and unpaid care for those with disabilities (which may involve evaluating the impact of encouraging greater work participation), and, of course, the best means of promoting and maintaining health in later life.

References

1. United Nations. World population prospects, the 2000 revision: Highlights. United Nations, New York, 2001.
2. OECD. Maintaining prosperity in an ageing society, Paris, OECD, 1999.
3. Grundy E. Gender and healthy ageing. In: *Longer Life and Healthy Ageing*, ed. Zeng Yi et al. Springer, 2006, 173–199.
4. Manton, K.G. and Gu, X. Changes in the prevalence of chronic disability in the United States black and nonblack population from age 65 from 1982 to 1999, *PNAS*, 98, 6354, 2001.
5. Sundström, G., Malmberg, B., and Johansson, L., Balancing family and state care: Neither, either or both? The case of Sweden, *Ageing Soc*, 26, 767, 2006.
6. Jacobzone, S., Cambois, E., Chaplain, E., and Robine J.M. Long term care services to older people, a perspective of future needs. The impact of an improving health of older persons, OECD, Paris. 1998.
7. Choi, N.G. Patterns and determinants of social service utilization: Comparison of the childless elderly and elderly parents living with or apart from their children, *Gerontologist*, 34(3), 353, 1994.
8. Sundström, G. Care by families: An overview of trends. In: Organisation for Economic Co-operation and Development, caring for frail elderly people, OECD, Paris, 1994.
9. Royal Commission on Long Term Care. With respect to old age: Long term care rights and responsibilities. Research vol. 1, *The Context of Long-Term Care Policy*, Cm 4192-II/1, The Stationery Office, London, 1999.
10. Broese van Groenou, M. et al. Socioeconomic status differences in the use of informal and formal help: A comparison of four European countries, *Ageing Soc*, 26, 745, 2006.

11. Goldscheider, F.K. and Waite, L.S. *New families, no families?* University of California Press, Berkeley, 1991.
12. Bath, P.A. and Deeg, D. Social engagement and health outcomes among older people: Introduction to a special section, *Eur J Ageing*, 2, 24, 2005.
13. Coleman, D. (ed.) *Europe's population in the 1990s*, Oxford University Press, Oxford, 1996, chap. 1.
14. Wolf, D.A. The elderly and their kin: Patterns of availability and access. In *Demography of Aging*, ed. Martin, L.G. and Preston, S.H. National Academy Press, Washington, D.C., 1994, 146.
15. Grundy, E. Demographic influences on the future of family care. In: *The Future of Family Care*, ed. Allen, I. and Perkins, E. HMSO, London, 1995, chap. 1.
16. Grundy, E. Population ageing in Europe. In: *Europe's Population in the 1990s*, ed. Coleman, D. Oxford University Press, Oxford, 1996, chap. 8.
17. Murphy, M. and Grundy, E. Mothers with living children and children with living mothers: The role of fertility and mortality in the period 1911–1950, *Population Trends*, 112, 36, 2003.
18. Murphy, M., Martikainen, P., and Pennec, S. Demographic change and the supply of potential family supporters in Britain, Finland and France in the period 1911–2050, *Eur J Population*, in press, 2006.
19. Grundy, E., Murphy, M., and Shelton, N. Looking beyond the household: Intergenerational perspectives on living kin and contacts with kin in Great Britain, *Population Trends*, 97, 19, 1999.
20. Henretta, J., Grundy, E., and Harris, S. Socioeconomic differences in having living parents and children, a US-British comparison of middle aged women, *J Marriage Family*, 63, 852, 2001.
21. Attias-Donfut, C., Ogg, J., and Wolff, F.C. European patterns of intergenerational financial and time transfers, *Eur J Ageing*, 2, 161, 2005.
22. Grundy, E. Reciprocity in relationships: Socioeconomic and health influences on intergenerational exchanges between third age parents and their adult children in Great Britain, *Br J Sociol*, 56, 233, 2005.
23. Elman, C. and Uhlenberg P. Co-residence in the early twentieth century: Elderly women in the United States and their children, *Population Stud*, 49, 501, 1995.
24. Grundy, E. and Murphy, M. Marital status and family support for the oldest old in Great Britain. In: *Human Longevity, Individual Life Duration, and the Growth of the Oldest-Old Population*, ed. Robine, J.-M., Crimmins, E.M., Horiuchi, S., and Zeng, Y. Springer, 2006, chap. 18.
25. Pampel, F.C. Trends in living alone among the elderly in Europe. In: *Elderly Migration and Population Redistribution*, ed. Rogers, A. Belhaven Press, London, 1992, chap. 6.
26. Grundy, E. The living arrangements of elderly people, *Rev Clin Gerontol* 2, 353, 1992.
27. Iacovou, M. Patterns of family living. In *Social Europe*, ed. Berthoud, R. and Iacovou, M. Edward Elgar, Cheltenham, 2004, chap. 2.
28. Tomassini, C. et al. Living arrangements among older people: An overview of trends in Europe and the USA, *Population Trends*, 115, 24, 2004.
29. Wolf, D. Changes in the living arrangements of older women: An international study, *Gerontologist*, 35, 724, 1995.
30. Choi, N.G. Racial differences in the determinants of the living arrangements of widowed and divorced elderly women, *Gerontologist*, 31, 496, 1991.

31. Clarke, C.J. and Neidert, L. Living arrangements of the elderly: An examination of differences according to ancestry and generation, *Gerontologist*, 32, 796, 1992.

32. Daatland, S.O. and Lowenstein, A. Intergenerational solidarity and the family-welfare state balance, *Eur J Ageing*, 2, 171, 2005.

33. Tomassini, C. et al., Contacts between elderly parents and their children in four European countries: Current patterns and future prospects, *Eur J Ageing*, 54, 63, 2004.

34. Hank, K., Proximity and contacts between older parents and their children: A European comparison. *J Marriage Family*, in press.

35. Janevic, M., Gjonca, E., and Hyde, M. *Physical and Social Environment in Health, Wealth and Lifestyles in the Older Population of England: The 2002 English Longitudinal Study of Ageing*, ed. Marmot, M. et al. The Institute for Fiscal Studies, London, 2003, 342.

36. Grundy, E. and Shelton, N. Contact between adult children and their parents in Great Britain 1986–1999, *Environ Planning*, 33, 685, 2001.

37. Henretta, J., Grundy, E., and Harris, S. The influence of socioeconomic and health differences on parents' provision of help to adult children: A British–United States comparison, *Ageing Soc*, 22, 441, 2002.

38. Lye, D.N., Klepinger, D.H., Davis, H.P., and Nelson, A. Childhood living arrangements and adult children's relations with their parents, *Demography*, 32, 261, 1995.

39. Ogg, J. and Renault, S. The support of parents in old age by those born during 1945–1954: A European perspective, *Ageing Soc*, 26, 723, 2006.

40. Bowling, A. and Grundy, E. The association between social networks and mortality in later life, *Rev Clin Gerontol*, 8, 353, 1998.

41. Grundy, E., Bowling, A., and Farquhar, M. Social support, life satisfaction and survival at older ages. In: *Health and Mortality among Elderly Populations*, ed. Caselli, G. and Lopez, A. Clarendon Press, Oxford, 1996, chap. 7.

42. Fratiglioni, L., Wang, H., and Ericsson, K. Influence of social networks on occurrence of dementia: A community-based longitudinal study, *Lancet*, 355, 1315, 2000.

43. Grundy, E. and Sloggett, A. Health inequalities in the older population: The role of personal capital, social resources and socioeconomic circumstances, *Soc Sci Med*, 56: 935, 2003.

44. Lyyra, T.M. and Heikkinen, R.L. Perceived social support and mortality in older people, *J Gerontol Soc Sci*, 61B, S147, 2006.

45. Antonucci, T.C., Arjouch, K.J., and Janevic, M.R. The effect of social relations with children on the education–health link in men and women aged 40 and over, *Soc Sci Med*, 56, 949, 2003.

46. Glass, T.A. et al. Population based study of social and productive activities as predictors of survival among elderly Americans, *BMJ*, 319, 478, 1999.

47. Glei, D.A. et al. Participating in social activities helps preserve cognitive function: An analysis of a longitudinal, population-based study of the elderly, *Int J Epidemiol*, 34, 864, 2005.

48. McIntyre, S. The effects of family position and status on health. *Soc Sci Med*, 35, 453, 1992.

49. Waite, L.J. Does marriage matter? *Demography*, 32, 483, 1995.

50. Goldman, N., Korenman, S., and Weinstein, R. Marital status and health among the elderly. *Soc Sci Med*, 40, 1717, 1995.

51. Wenger, G.C. *The Supportive Network: Coping with Old Age*, Allen and Unwin, London, 1984.
52. Lang, F.R. The availability and supportive functions of extended kinship ties in later life: Evidence from the Berlin Ageing Study. In: *Families in Ageing Societies*, ed. Harper, S. Oxford University Press, Oxford, 2004, chap. 4.
53. Barefoot, J.C. et al. Social network diversity and risks of ischemic heart disease and total mortality: Findings from the Copenhagen City Heart Study, *Am J Epidemiol*, 161, 960, 2005.
54. Netuveli, G. et al. Quality of life at older ages: Evidence from the English longitudinal study of ageing (wave 1), *J Epidemiol Community Health*, 60, 357, 2006.
55. Grundy, E. and Glaser, K. Trends in, and transitions to, institutional residence among older people in England and Wales, 1971 to 1991, *J Epidemiol Community Health*, 51, 531, 1997.
56. Carrière, Y, et al. Sociodemographic factors associated with the use of formal and informal support networks among elderly Canadians. In: *Longer Life and Healthy Ageing*, ed. Zeng, Y. et al. Springer, Dordrecht, 2006, chap. 17.
57. Grundy, E. et al. Living arrangements and place of death of older people with cancer in England and Wales: A record linkage study, *Br J Cancer*, 91, 907, 2004.
58. Grundy, E. Living arrangements and the health of older persons in developed countries. Population bulletin of the United Nations, special issue, living arrangements of older persons: Critical issues and policy responses, 42/43:311, 2001.
59. Sarwari, A.R. et al. Prospective study on the relation between living arrangement and change in functional health status of elderly women, *Am J Epidemiol*, 147, 370, 1998.
60. Kunemund, H. and Rein, M. There is more to giving than receiving: Theoretical arguments and empirical explorations of crowding in and crowding out, *Ageing Soc*, 19, 93, 1999.
61. Penning, M. and Keating, N. Self, informal and formal care: Partnerships in community based and residential long-term care settings, *Can J Aging*, 19, 75, 2000.
62. Bell, D. and Bowes, A. *Financial Care Models in Scotland and the UK*. Joseph Rowntree Foundation, York, 2006, 68.

chapter nine

Energy efficiency and the health of older people

Paul Wilkinson

Contents

Summary 103
Temperature and mortality in the United Kingdom 104
Pathophysiological mechanisms 105
The role of housing 106
Socioeconomic variations 110
Policy implications 112
References.. 113

Summary

It is now well recognised that older people are particularly vulnerable to adverse health effects from exposure to low and high ambient temperatures. In the United Kingdom, cold exposure appears to be the main factor contributing to the large burden of excess winter mortality, which in most years amounts to twenty thousand to fifty thousand deaths, the majority attributable to cardiovascular and respiratory disease.

An important mechanism for the winter increase in cardiovascular death appears to be changes to the circulation and haemostasis as a result of peripheral cooling and vasoconstriction. This may predispose to thrombotic events (myocardial infarction and strokes) in the context of pre-existing atherosclerosis.

Although exposure to cold through outdoor excursions may be important in precipitating cardiovascular deaths, there is now emerging evidence that people who live in inadequately heated homes of low energy efficiency are more vulnerable to winter- and cold-related mortality. They may also suffer a range of other adverse health effects, including detrimental impacts on psychosocial well-being. It appears, therefore, that appreciable health as well as environmental benefits can be expected from interventions aimed at improving the energy efficiency of the home.

Temperature and mortality in the United Kingdom

There is now a large body of evidence that older people are especially vulnerable to adverse health effects from exposure to low and high ambient temperatures [1,2]. Such evidence comes from a range of studies but, epidemiologically, it has been most clearly demonstrated by time-series regression studies that have examined the association between the daily fluctuation in mortality and outdoor temperature [3,4]. Such association is shown graphically for the London population aged sixty-five years or more in Figure 9.1. In panel (A), the daily counts of death and a one-month moving average of deaths are plotted against date for the period 2001–2003. The seasonality is very apparent, with the peak of deaths occurring during winter months. In most years, the one-month moving average of the daily death rates is found to be more than 40% higher at its winter peak than during the summer nadir. This is a remarkable degree of fluctuation given that it applies to all-cause deaths in the population as a whole.

To define the winter excess of mortality, it has become conventional to compare the death rates in the period from December to March with that observed in other months of the year. By this definition, the annual winter excess in the United Kingdom is usually between twenty thousand and fifty thousand deaths, with most of the excess attributable to deaths from cardiovascular and respiratory causes. Such an excess reflects a substantial burden, which has gained increasing attention in recent years. To put it into perspective, this number of deaths, even for an average winter in the United Kingdom, is at least as great, if not larger, than the number of deaths that occurred in France during the exceptional heat wave of 2003 (a 'one in five hundred years' event) [5].

The deaths in London during that same heat wave of 2003 are separately identified in the plots of Figure 9.1. It is clear that, compared with the normal summertime experience, the heat wave was associated with a very large—almost threefold—increase in deaths at its peak. Figure 9.1(B) illustrates the temperature dependence of mortality, after adjusting for seasonality and other time-varying risk factors. Daily mortality rises steadily at temperatures below a daily mean of about 18°C and also, more steeply, at mean temperatures above around 20°C. However, because there are many more cold days than hot, the total number of deaths attributable to the heat wave overall, which occurred over just a few days, was small by comparison with those due to cold. The official estimate of heat deaths during the heat wave of 2003 was in fact 2,091 for England and Wales [6,7], whilst the winter excess for the same year was at least ten times this figure.

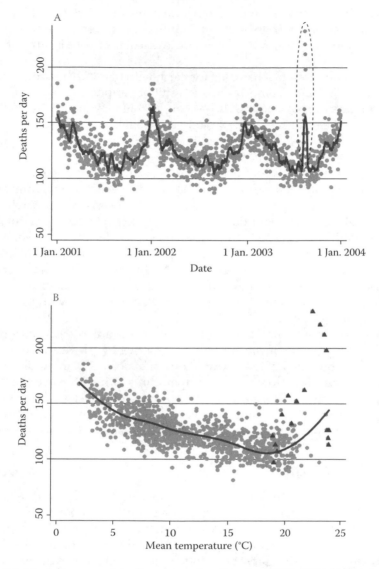

Figure 9.1 Mortality ages sixty-five years plus, London, 2001–2003. (A) against date and (B) against mean temperature of the preceding two weeks. Deaths occurring during the heat wave of August 2003 are circled (A) and shown as black triangles (B).

Pathophysiological mechanisms

Not all of the winter excess of deaths is due to cold, however. Winter respiratory infections such as influenza also often increase deaths during winter months, and in epidemic years, their impact can be very large. Other factors that contribute to the seasonal pattern may include behavioural changes, variations in micronutrient intake, and air pollution. Nonetheless, assessments that have examined the independent effect of cold in older people suggest that, in years without an influenza epidemic, between 50 and 60% of winter excess mortality from cardiovascular disease is attributable to cold [8,9].

The hypothesised mechanisms for cardiovascular death invoke changes to the circulation and haemostasis as a result of peripheral vascular constriction secondary to body cooling [10]—changes that may predispose to thrombotic events (heart attacks and stroke) [11]. Collins has also suggested that exposure to cold may directly affect the natural defences of the respiratory system to infection, which may therefore explain the rise in respiratory mortality, which tends to occur with a longer time-lag after cold exposure.

Collins and others have also provided evidence that behavioural as well as physiological changes may contribute to the increased vulnerability of older people in cold conditions. In a study comparing older men and younger adults, he observed that older people prefer the same room temperature (22–23°C) as young adults, but that they manipulated the temperature controls less precisely—suggesting that the threshold for a behavioural response to perceived discomfort due to cold is higher in older people [12]. There is also some evidence that ageing may be associated with progressive thermoregulatory impairment [13].

There is debate about whether the critical exposure to cold occurs during outdoor excursions or in the indoor environment [14]. Keatinge and colleagues have provided evidence in favour of exposure from outdoor excursions rather than from low indoor temperatures [4,15]. However, both may be important, and on theoretical grounds, it seems just as plausible that cooling from sitting in a cold indoor environment may have appreciably adverse effects, particularly on the circulatory system.

The role of housing

Pointers to the indoor environment and, specifically, to housing quality as important come from a number of directions. An often reported observation is that the United Kingdom has a larger winter excess of mortality than many other countries of continental Europe and Scandinavia [16], despite the fact that Britain is buffered against very cold winter temperatures by its maritime climate and the specific influence of the Gulf Stream. This seems paradoxical if cold is the principal factor contributing to excess winter death.

However, in part perhaps *because* of the mild winter temperatures in the United Kingdom, the housing stock has tended to be of comparatively poor thermal efficiency. In consequence, winter indoor temperatures can become very low [17]. This has been shown by measurements of indoor temperatures made by automatic data loggers in dwellings awaiting energy efficiency upgrades as part of England's national energy efficiency programme (*Warm Front*): many homes have standardised day-time living room temperatures and/or night-time bedroom temperatures below 16°C when the maximum outdoor temperature is below 5°C [18].

Moreover, such measurements have demonstrated the relationship between standardised indoor temperature during cold weather and the energy efficiency rating of the dwelling (Figure 9.2). The horizontal axis of Figure 9.2 is the standard assessment procedure (SAP) scale, which is a measure of the space and hot water heating cost normalised for floor area, assuming a standard heating pattern. It is fixed on a semilogarithmic scale resulting in a range for SAP scores between 0 (least energy efficient) and 120 (most energy efficient) [19]. The heating cost is calculated using a modified degree day method to take account of incidental gains. The average SAP rating of a English dwelling in 2001 is estimated as 48 and a new dwelling built to the 2001 building regulations has a SAP of around 75 [20]. As might be expected, the curves show that heating costs and carbon dioxide emissions increase as the SAP rating falls, and standardised temperatures fall as well. Lower energy efficiency is also associated with higher standardised relative humidity and mould growth [21].

The importance of these observations is that emerging evidence suggests that indoor temperature is an important determinant of cold-related mortality and morbidity, primarily for cardiovascular disease (Table 9.1 and Figure 9.3). The data of Table 9.1 show the results of a study that linked daily mortality data, 1986–1996, to the 1991 English House Conditions Survey using the postcode of residence [17]. It is clear from this data that excess winter death (here using the December to March comparison with other months) is strongly aligned to age, rising to 30% by the 85+ age group. It is also slightly greater in women than men for reasons that do not appear to be related to differences in age or medical status [8]. However, arguably the most important observation is the apparently strong association between the magnitude of the winter excess risk and property age.

To a large degree, the age of a property determines the standard and fabric of the dwelling and thus its energy efficiency. The older the dwelling is, the poorer its energy efficiency and (in general) the colder the winter indoor temperatures. The trend of a declining risk of winter death with more recent build appears quite robust and is most readily interpreted as a reflection of indoor temperatures. This conclusion is further supported by the (less clear) statistical trend for the risk of excess winter death to be greater in the coolest dwellings.

Recent analyses have shown a gradual decline in temperature-related deaths over the course of the twentieth century, despite an ageing population (Figure 9.4) [22]. Such analyses cannot identify the specific factors contributing to this decline, but the trend is likely to reflect improvements in a range of social, environmental, behavioural, and health care factors, including housing quality. However, although the burdens of cold-related death have diminished substantially, they remain large, and the fact that there has been a decline, points to modifiable factors that may offer the potential for further reduction in cold-related mortality burdens.

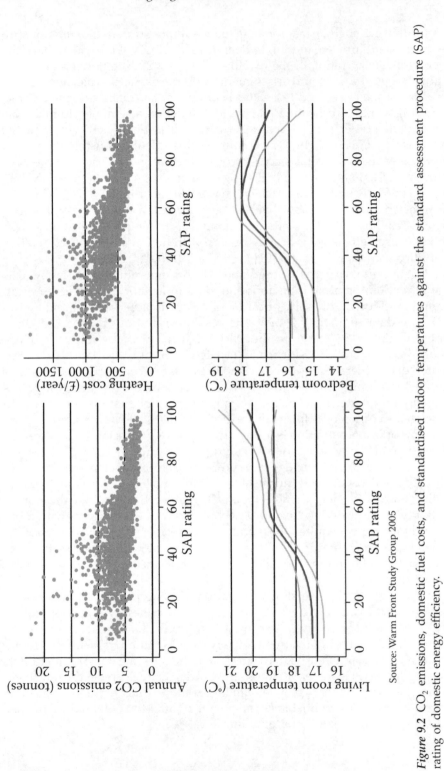

Figure 9.2 CO$_2$ emissions, domestic fuel costs, and standardised indoor temperatures against the standard assessment procedure (SAP) rating of domestic energy efficiency.

Source: Warm Front Study Group 2005

Table 9.1 Excess Winter Death from Cardiovascular Disease, England, 1986–1996

	Winter deaths	% Excess in winter	Risk (95% CI) relative to baseline	P-value
Age-group (*n* = 80,331)				
0–44	385	1.3	1.0	
45–64	4,008	18.9	1.17 (1.03–1.34)	
65–74	16,619	21.0	1.20 (1.05–1.36)	<0.001
75–84	23,204	22.6	1.21 (1.07–1.38)	
85+	14,169	30.0	1.28 (1.13–1.46)	
Sex (n = 80,331)				
Male	15,000	21.3	1.0	
Female	15,467	24.5	1.03 (1.02–1.05)	0.09
SEG, head of household (*n* = 37,700)				
Professional	580	31.3	1.0	
Managerial	2,251	25.5	0.96 (0.85–1.07)	
Intermed nonmanual	1,197	21.8	0.93 (0.82–1.05)	
Junior nonmanual	1,447	25.1	0.95 (0.84–1.08)	>0.2
Skilled manual	4,831	22.6	0.93 (0.84–1.04)	
Semiskilled	2,803	23.3	0.94 (0.84–1.05)	
Unskilled	1,238	21.3	0.92 (0.82–1.05)	
Property age (*n* = 80,331)				
Before 1850	701	28.2	1.0	
1850–1899	5,469	25.6	0.98 (0.88–1.09)	
1900–1918	3,063	24.1	0.97 (0.87–1.08)	
1919–1944	6,978	26.0	0.98 (0.89–1.09)	0.001
1945–1964	6,709	23.9	0.97 (0.87–1.07)	
1965–1980	6,612	17.1	0.91 (0.82–1.01)	
After 1980	935	15.0	0.90 (0.79–1.02)	
Indoor temp. index (*n* = 14,739)				
Quartile 1 (warmest)	1,498	13.4	1.0	
Quartile 2	1,357	26.5	1.11 (1.02–1.22)	0.002
Quartile 3	1,247	17.5	1.04 (0.94–1.14)	
Quartile 4 (coolest)	1,488	36.3	1.20 (1.09–1.32)	

Note: Based on analysis of mortality records linked to the 1991 English House Condition Survey.

Source: Adapted from Wilkinson, P. et al., *Cold comfort: The social and environmental determinants of excess winter death in England, 1986–1996*. York: Joseph Rowntree Foundation, 2001.

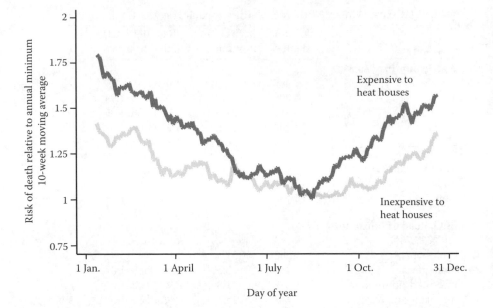

Figure 9.3 Seasonal variation in deaths from cardiovascular disease by standardized cost of home heating, England, 1986–1996. (From Wilkinson, P. et al., *Cold comfort: The social and environmental determinants of excess winter death in England, 1986–1996.* York: Joseph Rowntree Foundation, 2001.)

Socioeconomic variations

Interestingly, Table 9.1 shows *no* gradient in risk with socioeconomic status, despite the fact that deprivation is a strong predictor of death rates overall, especially from cardiovascular disease. In fact, this lack of socioeconomic gradient has been a consistent finding in the United Kingdom [8,23] and elsewhere [24]. If there is a gradient of risk with socioeconomic status, the balance of evidence suggests that it is small.

This observation appears at odds with the notion that indoor temperature is the critical factor for winter death, as it is generally assumed that those on low incomes are least able to afford to heat the home to an adequate temperature and would thus be most vulnerable. This has led to the concept of fuel poverty. A household is said to be fuel poor if it needs to spend more than 10% of its income on fuel in order to maintain adequate space heating.

However, we have previously shown that, in fact, lower socioeconomic groups do not *on average* have cooler homes than higher socioeconomic groups. This observation may reflect behavioural influences, but also the fact that housing association and local authority dwellings are often heated as well as or better than owner-occupied dwellings [17]. This partly reflects the relatively recent year of construction of much social housing and the efforts by local authorities to ensure energy efficiency in their housing stock. Poverty *is* associated with poorer home heating when heating costs are high. The

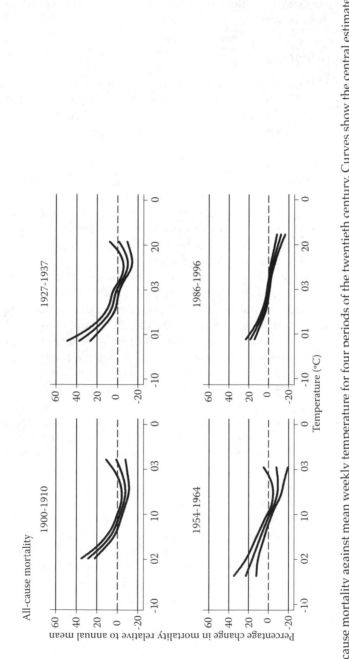

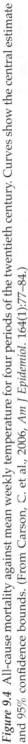

Figure 9.4 All-cause mortality against mean weekly temperature for four periods of the twentieth century. Curves show the central estimate and 95% confidence bounds. (From Carson, C. et al., 2006, *Am J Epidemiol.* 164(1):77–84.)

lack of socioeconomic gradient in risk therefore appears compatible with a temperature-related impact.

Policy implications

The influence of inadequate home heating on the risk of cold-related death has not been widely tested [15]. However, the limited evidence available suggests a probable link that has a strong theoretical plausibility: older people in particular spend a great deal of their time at home indoors, and their temperature environments often appear to be sufficiently cold to have appreciable physiological effects on the circulation and blood. Moreover, we know that there are other, well-documented adverse effects on health and well-being of living in a cold environment. We know also that improvements in energy efficiency help to increase indoor temperatures, and the experience from England is that such improvements reduce the occurrence of dampness and mould, which have their own health effects [25–28], without compromising ventilation characteristics of the dwelling [29].

These favourable changes to the indoor environment can be expected to have a range of health benefits, particularly for older people. Assessment of impacts on mortality remains indirect and dependent on assumptions of causality from the epidemiological evidence. But there is more direct evidence of psychosocial benefits. Recipients of the *Warm Front* energy efficiency improvements, for example, reported a wide range of apparent benefits, ranging from thermal comfort; satisfaction with improved and more controllable warmth/hot water; perceptions of improved physical health and comfort, especially of mental and emotional well-being; improved family relations; expansion of the domestic space used during cold months; increased privacy within the home; and improved social interaction [30].

A potentially important but so far unquantified influence of energy efficiency improvement is its contribution to the alleviation of poverty. The potential cost savings may be particularly important for those on low income, which of course includes many people above retirement age. However, it appears that many lower income households choose to take the benefits of improved energy efficiency through warmer indoor temperatures rather than as reduced fuel bills. Whether this is the case for other households is not clear, and whether this may change given the recent steep rises in fuel costs remains to be seen. However, at present, it appears the main benefit of energy efficiency is through its influence on temperature.

Overall, the evidence appears sufficient to conclude that appreciable health benefits would accrue from interventions that improve the energy efficiency of dwellings. Arguably, it is also preferable to try to upgrade the thermal efficiency of properties rather than, say, giving winter fuel allowances to older people. Greater thermal efficiency should guarantee warmer and better controlled indoor temperatures, whilst a fuel allowance can always be spent on other things (including Christmas presents for grandchildren!). The case in favour of energy efficiency interventions is made easier because they are comparatively inexpensive and can be supported on environmental and/or cost grounds. If the gain in energy efficiency is taken as lower fuel bills, the average saving per year in standardised fuel costs is estimated to offset the capital expenditure required for a typical energy efficiency upgrade within around ten years. As just observed, however, some households choose to take at least part of the efficiency saving as a warmer indoor environment rather than cost saving. The health benefits related to temperature increase appear to compare favourably with many forms of health care interventions.

It is worth noting that the problem of winter indoor cold appears to be widely distributed in the population, and it is the older people who are most vulnerable. Thus, whilst initiatives to target the fuel poor are welcome, there is also a need to raise the energy efficiency standard of new and existing housing stock more generally. In this regard, it is very welcome that the Home Health and Safety Rating System [31] incorporates an assessment of the adequacy of energy efficiency in health terms and that higher energy efficiency standards are being incorporated into new building regulation. However, the case seems strong for public policies that will further enhance the energy efficiency of new and existing housing stock in Britain.

References

1. Goodwin J. Cold stress. Circulatory illness and the elderly. In: *Cutting the cost of cold*, ed. Rudge J, Nicol F. London: E&FN Spon, 2000.
2. Keatinge WR. Winter mortality and its causes. *Int J Circumpolar Health*. 2002, 61(4):292–299.
3. Braga AL, Zanobetti A, Schwartz J. The effect of weather on respiratory and cardiovascular deaths in 12 U.S. cities. *Environ Health Perspect*. 2002, 110(9):859–863.
4. The Eurowinter Group. Cold exposure and winter mortality from ischaemic heart disease, cerebrovascular disease, respiratory disease, and all causes in warm and cold regions of Europe. *Lancet*. 1997, 349(9062):1341–1346.
5. Le Tertre A, Lefranc A, Eilstein D, Declercq C, Medina S, Blanchard M, et al. Impact of the 2003 heat wave on all-cause mortality in 9 French cities. *Epidemiology*. 2006, 17(1):75–79.
6. Johnson H, Kovats RS, McGregor G, Stedman J, Gibbs M, Walton H, et al. The impact of the 2003 heat wave on mortality and hospital admissions in England. *Health Stat Q*. 2005, Spring (25):6–11.
7. Stedman J. The predicted number of air pollution related deaths in the U.K. during the August 2003 heat wave. *Atmospheric Environ*. 2004, 38(8):1087–1090.
8. Wilkinson P, Pattenden S, Armstrong B, Fletcher A, Kovats RS, Mangtani P, et al. Vulnerability to winter mortality in elderly people in Britain: Population-based study. *Br Med J*. 2004, 329(7467):647.
9. Armstrong B, Wilkinson P, Stevenson S. Identifying components of seasonal variation in mortality. *Epidemiology*. 2000, 11(4):S113.
10. Smolander J. Effect of cold exposure on older humans. *Int J Sports Med*. 2002, 23(2):86–92.

11. Woodhouse PR, Khaw KT, Plummer M. Seasonal variation of blood pressure and its relationship to ambient temperature in an elderly population. *J Hypertens*. 1993, 11(11):1267–1274.

12. Collins KJ, Exton-Smith AN, Dore C. Urban hypothermia: preferred temperature and thermal perception in old age. *Br Med J (Clin Res Ed)*. 1981, 282(6259):175–177.

13. Collins KJ, Dore C, Exton-Smith AN, Fox RH, MacDonald IC, Woodward PM. Accidental hypothermia and impaired temperature homoeostasis in the elderly. *Br Med J*. 1977, 1(6057):353–356.

14. Goodwin J, Taylor RS, Pearce VR, Read KL. Seasonal cold, excursional behaviour, clothing protection and physical activity in young and old subjects. *Int J Circumpolar Health*. 2000, 59(3–4):195–203.

15. Keatinge WR, Coleshaw SR, Holmes J. Changes in seasonal mortalities with improvement in home heating in England and Wales from 1964 to 1984. *Int J Biometeorol*. 1989, 33(2):71–76.

16. Mercer JB. Cold—An underrated risk factor for health. *Environ Res*. 2003, 92(1):8–13.

17. Wilkinson P, Landon M, Armstrong B, Stevenson S, McKee M. *Cold comfort: The social and environmental determinants of excess winter death in England, 1986–1996*. York: Joseph Rowntree Foundation, 2001.

18. Oreszczyn T, Hong S, Ridley I, Wilkinson P, for the Warm Front Study Group. Determinants of winter indoor temperatures in low income households in England. Energy Buildings. 2006, 38(3):245–252.

19. BRECSU (on behalf of DEFRA). The Government's Standard Assessment Procedure for Energy Rating of Dwellings, Version 9.70, 2001 edition Garston, Watford: BRE, 2001.

20. Shorrock L, Utley J. Domestic energy fact file 2003 (BR 457), Watford: BRE; 2003.

21. Oreszczyn T, Ridley I, Hong SH, Wilkinson P. Mould and winter indoor relative humidity in low income households in England. Indoor built environment. *Indoor Built Environ*. 2006, 15(2):125–135.

22. Carson C, Hajat S, Armstrong B, Wilkinson P. Declining vulnerability to temperature-related mortality in London over the 20th century. *Am J Epidemiol*. 2006, 164(1):77–84.

23. Aylin P, Morris S, Wakefield J, Grossinho A, Jarup L, Elliott P. Temperature, housing, deprivation and their relationship to excess winter mortality in Great Britain, 1986–1996. *Int J Epidemiol*. 2001, 30(5):1100–1108.

24. Rau R. Winter mortality in elderly people in Britain: Lack of social gradient in winter excess mortality is obvious in Denmark. *Br Med J*. 2004, 329(7472):976–977.

25. Howden-Chapman P. Housing standards: A glossary of housing and health. *J Epidemiol Community Health*. 2004, 58(3):162–168.

26. Bornehag CG, Sundell J, Bonini S, Custovic A, Malmberg P, Skerfving S, et al. Dampness in buildings as a risk factor for health effects, EUROEXPO: A multidisciplinary review of the literature (1998–2000) on dampness and mite exposure in buildings and health effects. *Indoor Air*. 2004, 14(4):243–257.

27. Evans J, Hyndman S, Stewart-Brown S, Smith D, Petersen S. An epidemiological study of the relative importance of damp housing in relation to adult health. *J Epidemiol Community Health*. 2000, 54(9):677–686.

28. Peat JK, Dickerson J, Li J. Effects of damp and mould in the home on respiratory health: A review of the literature. *Allergy.* 1998, 53(2):120–128.

29. Manuel J. A healthy home environment? *Environ Health Perspect.* 1999, 107(7):A352–357.

30. Gilbertson J, Stevens M, Stiell B, Thorogood N. Home is where the hearth is: grant recipients' views of England's home energy efficiency scheme (Warm Front). *Soc Sci Med.* 2006, 63(4):946–956.

31. ODPM. Statistical evidence to support the housing health and safety rating system. Vols 1–3: Project report, summary of results and technical appendix. London: Office of the Deputy Prime Minister, May 2003.

chapter ten

Ageing, health, and welfare: an economic perspective

Charles Normand

Contents

Introduction 117
Ageing and work 118
Ageing and caring 120
Ageing and needs for health and social care 121
The pension issue 122
Financial versus economic perspectives 124
Concluding comments 125
References 126

Introduction

Prediction of dire consequences of population ageing for the economies of Western countries is common [1], despite long-standing evidence that changes are likely to be gradual and the effect complex [2–4]. The range of concerns includes an increasing dependency ratio (that is, a higher proportion of the population that is not engaged in paid work), a shortage of workers for a wide range of jobs, higher costs for pensions and other income transfers, a shortage of people to provide paid and unpaid caring, and higher costs for health and social care. Whilst it is true that the changing population structure will have important economic impacts, there is reason to believe that the changes can be accommodated without the more serious problems cited.

In some cases the analysis fails to understand the underlying economic principles, and all too often the analysis ignores important insights from policy-relevant research such as the effects of ageing on patterns of health service use [5]. Much of the concern also stems from a belief that conventions such as the age for retirement have some underlying logic rather than being social artefacts. Current arrangements for providing income in old age can make it difficult to continue to work without financial penalties, and the resulting incentives may deter people from useful paid work.

The emerging debate about retirement has produced some useful ideas, but structures and rules still make gradual and phased retirement difficult. 'Early retirement' as a form of workforce management was common in the 1980s and 1990s and, in many organisations, the cost of workforce restructuring was transferred to pension schemes (putting further pressure on their liquidity). In many countries, unemployment in the workforce was high in these periods, and there were advantages politically (and for many employers) to shifting the unemployment into the older parts of the population (and rebranding it as retirement). At least some parts of the challenge of the ageing population can be accommodated by making better use of the available population of people willing and able to work.

Ageing and work

It is common, where people have the choice, for work of some sort to continue long past the conventional retirement ages of sixty or sixty-five. The current number of individuals working in the United Kingdom past age sixty-five is around 582,000, and this is projected to rise to 775,000 by 2020 [6]. This suggests that the proportion of the population over sixty-five in paid work will remain fairly constant at around 6%. What this disguises is that the proportion of people aged between sixty-five and sixty-nine in employment would be expected to rise. Between 2006 and 2020 there is likely to be a rise of only 10% in the numbers between sixty-five and sixty-nine; the population over sixty-five in total will rise by 29% [7]. For obvious reasons, the largest pool of potential additional workers will come from the younger elderly rather than the older old, so the rise in the potential workforce will be limited by the relatively small rise in those between sixty-five and sixty-nine.

It is hard to find the origins of the idea that people should retire at sixty or sixty-five. In 1981 a male of sixty-five had a life expectancy of around thirteen years, and this is likely to rise to around seventeen years in 2006 and twenty years by 2020. Put another way, a person retiring at seventy in 2020 would have a longer retirement than a person retiring at sixty-five in 1981. Evidence on compression of morbidity (and therefore the likelihood that a person of a given age will be fit to work) is a bit mixed [8], but this significant rise in life expectancy is probably associated with better general health for the 'younger old' and therefore their ability to work. The current pool of potential workers between sixty-five and sixty-nine is around 2.5 million for the United Kingdom, and this will rise to more than 3 million by 2020. This represents a considerable resource.

Of course many people do not want to continue to work, and many people have sufficient resources to stop work at or before the age of sixty-five. However, it is interesting to look at the current incentives to work for those of age sixty-five and above. For those in final salary pension schemes, there can be serious constraints to moving to a lower paid job, even within the same organisation, since this can reduce the value of pensions. Some pension schemes allow continued work, but for many the choice to continue work is a choice effectively to work for half pay, since the opportunity cost of not taking the pension can be up to half the salary. The decision to work and not take the pension increases income by half, but this is at the expense of having to continue full-time work. Some account of this problem is being taken with more flexible rules on work for those on state pensions, and in some cases people are able to draw some part of occupational pensions whilst working full (or nearly full) time. However, for many people the decision to remain in paid employment is essentially a decision to work for half pay.

In general there tend to be constraints on moving from higher to lower paid employment within the same organisation. Given that senior jobs are increasingly stressful, it is quite understandable that a person will choose not to continue in such a role, but that the person might quite happily resume a previous role. A good example of this is the way that, in the Roman Catholic Church, it is common for retired parish priests to resume work as curates. In academic work, it is common for a person to step down from roles as dean or department head whilst remaining active in teaching and research. After retirement, many academics continue to work for little or no pay in honorary or emeritus roles.

In manual jobs, the constraint to continue full-time work can be physical, but there are many jobs that are well within the physical strength of many people in their late sixties. For some the option to continue work would be attractive so long as the job was within their physical capability. Given that most manual jobs do not require great strength, it should in general be possible to offer people jobs well past age sixty-five if that is what they want.

Those who work for themselves have the option to retire gradually, and many take this route out of the labour force. This allows responsibility to be passed gradually to new managers or owners. In family businesses, this is particularly common as children gradually take over control from parents. It seems that, where people have a choice, a proportion opts to retire slowly and to reduce their work effort (and associated income) over a transitional period. In particular, in cases where the incentives are largely neutral, people seem to choose to continue to work but usually to a decreasing extent as time goes on.

The two main concerns expressed about the effect of ageing on the economy are the decrease in the number of workers and the increase in the number of nonworkers. It can be seen that changing the incentives and structures around retirement can potentially reduce these potential problems by having a larger proportion of the population employed. The ways to achieve this are likely to include changes in rules over incomes and pensions, changes in employment rules and practices to allow the choice of continued work with less stress and responsibility, and flexible approaches to allow work patterns that fit the needs of older workers.

Two other factors can reduce the economic impact of ageing. First, labour productivity can increase to allow increased output even with a falling number of workers. Productivity growth is in some senses exogenous (i.e., new ideas and inventions emerge over time) but, to some extent, the driver of productivity growth is necessity. As the population of working age falls and as this starts to put upward pressure on wage levels, new ideas are developed and put into effect. The international differences in labour productivity show that there are more efficient methods that are not adopted, especially in countries that have surplus labour.

In addition to new techniques and technology, new ideas about how to use these can have a profound effect. A simple example is the technology of cardiac surgery. Although some equipment has emerged, to a large extent the basic techniques in coronary artery bypass surgery have remained very similar, but the times spent intubated have fallen and the stay in hospital has become shorter, so the costs have fallen significantly. It seems to take time for people to learn how to exploit new technologies to best effect, and in some cases the full effects are delayed many years. These different forms of productivity growth have, in the past, been part of the cause of high unemployment, but with a labour shortage, measures to improve labour productivity can be part of the solution.

Second, despite the early effects of demographic change, in many countries in Western Europe unemployment remains high, particularly in Central and Eastern Europe. To an extent, the problems of a declining workforce may be the solution to unemployment. Of course, even with very high levels of employment there are people unsuited to the available vacancies, and an implication of a declining population of working age is the need to improve education and training opportunities to improve the match of available workers and vacant posts.

Whilst it is clearly the case that population ageing will reduce the proportion of the population in the conventional working age categories, the various points discussed here suggest that the problems will arise quite slowly. With a longer working life, lower unemployment, and measures to increase productivity, it may be possible to accommodate the changes with little difficulty.

Ageing and caring

In the previous section the general issue of retirement and the proportion of the workforce that is not employed was discussed. Since people tend to remain in good health long past the conventional retirement age, it is clear that many in the potential pool of workers are interested in at least some work. In a similar way, whilst the number of old (and particularly very old) people is increasing the need for care, the increase in the population of older people is increasing the number of potential carers.

This is not a straightforward story. A key issue is how many older people in the future will be living alone and how many will be in households with two or more people. Patterns of marriage and life expectancy are all contributing to an increase in the number of older couples, although there is some uncertainty how this will be affected by future patterns of divorce. Overall, it is likely that, although the absolute number of older people living alone will increase, proportionately there is likely to be a trend towards more older-age couples. The current situation is that more than half of women seventy-five and over live alone whilst in this age group only a third of men live alone [9]. As life expectancy for men rises more rapidly than for women, it is reasonable to expect that there will be a higher proportion of households with two or more people in this age category.

In many cases couples who each have disabilities care for each other. The key requirement is that between the two there is sufficient capacity to remain independent over the main living tasks. In many cases, it is necessary only to have one competent person for any given task so that viable couples may have complementary skills. If the number of older couples increases, it is likely that between them there will be disabilities that limit capacities to carry out daily living tasks, but that these can be overcome. Taking this into account means that it may be possible for couples to remain in home settings for longer with the need for only modest support despite the presence of disabilities.

From the point of view of the economic impact of ageing, the key point of this section is that increasing numbers of older people provide a caring resource as well as an increase in needs for care. This is not to say that the overall need for care will not increase, but the increased need will be met, to some extent, by more carers in the older population.

Ageing and needs for health and social care

A large part of the concern about population ageing is the perception that this will lead to a large increase in costs of health and social care [10]. Once again the evidence suggests that this is likely to be a more complicated picture. In brief, the need for hospital services is likely to increase only slightly, but the need for social and nursing care is likely to rise more significantly. Studies show that the pressure is more likely to come from demands to treat older people better, rather than from the increased numbers of older people [3].

The reason for the quite modest increase in costs of acute hospital care is mainly the key role of proximity to death in determining costs. It is now well established that much of the ill health that leads to high use of hospital services occurs in the last months of life [5,11,12]. Simple scaling up on the basis of age and gender utilisation patterns ignores this key point. If proximity to death costs is taken into account, the annual rise in acute care costs that is likely from the pure effects of population ageing is likely to be around 2% for the United Kingdom [13]. Put another way, this increase is likely to be below the rate of economic growth and therefore the capacity of countries to afford the care.

Part of the reason why the increase is quite slow is that costs of care in the last year of life fall with age. It is easy to understand why this might be the case. Take the example of lung cancer, which has very poor survival at all ages. Despite this, the patterns show that much more effort is made to intervene in younger people with lung cancer, and every effort is made to effect a cure. In the case of older people, the decision to treat the case as palliative occurs earlier. In some cases, this also reflects the presence of other illnesses in older people that make it less likely that treatment will be effective. The cost of the acute care near the end of life can fall by up to a third when compared to deaths in younger people, even when diagnosis is taken into account.

A reasonable criticism of this type of study is that it models the increased costs on the basis of retaining the current inequalities in access to care. There is increasing evidence of age and social class barriers to care, only some of which can be explained by relevant factors such as other morbidities. However, the important point is that ageing in itself represents only a modest driver of the pattern of acute care costs.

Whilst the evidence is clear that acute care costs will rise only modestly, the need for social and nursing care, particularly to support living at home, is likely to rise rapidly. Work in this area is constrained by the lack of good databases, but it seems again that social rather than medical care will rise the most. What is striking is that social care costs rise rapidly as death approaches, and costs are much higher for people who die old. This means that the ageing of the population is likely to lead to very large increases in the costs of social and nursing care. However, this must be seen in context. Costs for these elements of care are currently much less than for acute care (typically between 10 and 20%), so the high proportionate increases in costs will not translate into much higher overall costs.

The pension issue

An important driver of the current panic about population ageing is the supposed burden of pension costs [14]. Projections of these costs are causing serious reappraisal of policy in the United States, and there are constant reminders in Europe of the scale of liabilities to pay pensions. In the private sector, this is manifest as firms with deficits in their pension funds, and in some cases the pension deficit exceeds the value of firms. It is interesting to reflect that, in some cases in the 1980s and early 1990s, pension funds were considered to be overfunded, and contribution holidays were allowed or contribution rates reduced.

The pension 'problem' stems largely from the increased number of people who are likely to be alive past the age of sixty-five. It has already been suggested that combinations of generally higher retirement ages and increased wage income for those over sixty-five may reduce the need for transfers from the working to the nonworking population. A further source of potential saving is in the reduction of young dependents. It is estimated by the government actuary that there will be a fall of over 4% in the number of people age twenty and under by 2020, so, to an extent, the increase in nonworking elderly will be offset by a decrease in nonworking young. The number of people over age sixty-five is likely to rise by 2.8 million and the number age twenty and under will fall by 625,000—a net increase of 2.2 million in those in age groups that are typically not employed. Whilst it is true that support for younger people does not typically involve formal transfers from the working population, the overall burden on the working population depends on all categories of nonworkers. If we combine those age twenty and under and those sixty-five and over, the ratio of nonworkers to workers will rise from 0.72 in 2006 to 0.74 in 2020.

In a formal sense, the problem of pensions and the problem of paying for care for older people are similar. In both cases people need to transfer rights to funds across time. During the period in which people are earning more than they need to live, they save and hope to get back this saving in the form of income security and access to services in older age. Intertemporal transfers of rights are always difficult to enforce. There are many examples of governments, financial institutions, firms, and individuals reneging on commitments. For example, the inflation in the 1970s effectively transferred assets from lenders to borrowers, thereby reducing the value of previous savings. There have been many well publicised cases of company pension schemes failing to pay the full pension (and in some cases pay little or nothing), and the recent case of Equitable Life shows that even well established pension companies can fail significantly to meet their promises to pensioners. The role of government as a regulator in pensions reflects the difficulty in ensuring that promises are met. Governments in many countries are trying to shift responsibility for saving onto individuals so as to reduce government liability to pay future pensions. Experience suggests that, for this to succeed, strong regulation and probably some government backing to insuring or guaranteeing these schemes will be needed.

The mechanism by which rights to resources are transferred over time is mainly to use the savings to buy assets, and the combination of realising these assets and returns from the assets allows previous savers to become net spenders. For example, savings might be used to buy office or factory buildings, which are rented to businesses. This rent and the sale of such assets can allow pensions to be paid. This works well when interest rates and rents are high, since this provides a good return on savings and good pensions. It works less well when returns are low, since this means that more has to be saved to ensure a pension is paid in full. Returns in the 1980s and early 1990s tended to be well above historical patterns and led to a belief that pensions could be funded by this mechanism. More recent experience has been of returns well below the historical patterns, and it has been difficult for pension funds to meet commitments. This has been made worse by some pessimistic forecasts of life expectancy, which has risen in a linear path in recent years. Thus, poor returns on savings and longer than expected survival have combined to create a pension 'crisis'.

Generally, there is little reason to be worried by the current difficulties in the pensions industry. Just as it was unwise to expect the high returns to persist, it is unwise to expect the current low returns to continue. However, if there is a large shift towards personal saving to fund retirement there is a reason to believe that returns will remain depressed, since interest rates are the price of savings, and if savings increase, interest rates are likely to fall. Put another way, if we save too much it becomes difficult to find productive ways to invest such savings. Given the increasing globalisation in capital markets, such effects might be quite modest for individual countries; nevertheless, if savings were to increase significantly across developed countries there could be overall impacts on returns.

Savings and the purchase of assets on behalf of savers provide a mechanism to allow nonworking people to enjoy a share of national income. In effect, the working population consumes less and the nonworking population consumes more. Working people borrow money to fund house purchases (and other purchases) and pay interest and repayments to those who previously saved. The other way in which significant funds are transferred from the working to the nonworking population is through tax and public spending. It is now becoming clear that to pay pensions at the rates previously promised to people over the current retirement age is likely to require savings as well as tax mechanisms. Tax transfers do not have a direct effect on capital markets, such as the potential effect of depressing interest rates, and may also be needed to fund pensions for those who did not have sufficient funds to save during their working lives.

Financial versus economic perspectives

Economists make the distinction between costs and transfer payments. A cost is a use of resources to produce goods and services, whilst a transfer payment simply shifts spending power between individuals. When a parent gives a child pocket money, this does not make the family richer or poorer (at least not initially). Similarly, taxation used to make payments of pensions and other benefits does not make the country richer or poorer, but simply redistributes spending power between individuals. In that sense, government spending on pensions is not a cost and will not have the same macroeconomic effects as spending on building roads or paying teachers. This is not to say that transfer payments have no economic effects, since the change of who can spend will normally affect how the money is eventually used. Whilst government spending on goods and services effectively displaces private spending on goods and services, transfer payments simply redistribute the right to spend.

The desire of government to control public expenditure has several motivations, including the desire to avoid forcing voters to pay more tax, a desire to allow people to make their own choices on how to spend, and a desire to increase economic growth (which may be increased by shifting to more productive investments). It is not clear that tax that pays pensions has significant macroeconomic effects, so the main concern is the unpopularity of tax amongst those who pay. When a government claims the country cannot afford to pay higher pensions, it is really saying that those able to pay higher taxes are not willing to do so, and it is politically difficult to force them to do so. Ultimately, the issue is not really how we fund pensions, but to what extent the working population is willing to support the nonworking population. Private pensions and those based on previous saving transfer resources through giving nonworking people rights to own assets that can be exploited for their value in use or sale. This may be more acceptable to the working population and may have some macroeconomic advantages, but ultimately the two groups in the population are competing for the current resources, and gains to one group will be made mainly at the expense of the other.

Concluding comments

Given that population ageing is, to an extent, the triumph of public health, it is sad that the consequences so often produce gloomy comments. The overall argument from the different aspects of ageing discussed here is that this gloom is largely misplaced. Of course, there will be important changes to accommodate and some costs will rise, but none of these should be difficult to manage in a growing economy.

In some respects, it is not the growing number of older people, but rather the growing expectations of older people that will be hard to accommodate. Age discrimination in access to effective treatments is becoming less acceptable, and many of the successes of medical developments provide treatments of particular value to older people. Older people will form larger parts of the voting population, and there are already signs that people are willing to use voting power.

Some traditions are likely to be the victims of population ageing, especially final salary pension schemes (as currently constituted) and the right to retire whilst still fit and able to work. The interaction of work-related income and pension income to provide financial stability in older age will change, and it will become easier to choose a slower and more flexible shift from full-time work to not working. Pensions will be affordable, but those able to work are more likely to do so. Nothing removes the inherent tension between the desires of the working and the nonworking populations to have higher incomes, and the underlying dilemma is not resolved simply by shifting responsibility to individuals to save more. It is increasingly clear that government will play a larger role in the pension system, even if this is as a regulator and guarantor rather than as a funder.

The need for care will rise but so too will the pool of carers. The main risk is the likely failure to foresee the changing patterns of need rather than the absolute level of need for health and social care. Ageing will lead to much more need for nonhospital care, and the balance of needs will change. Perhaps the most important thing is to embrace the complexity of the effects of ageing. There will not be a crisis and ageing will come to be seen as a triumph of health and social policies, but some of the solutions are complex, and polices will have to recognise this.

References

1. http://news.scotsman.com/latest.cfm?id=2116812005 (accessed 02/08/06).
2. Raleigh VS. The demographic timebomb. *BMJ* 1997, 315:442–443.
3. Barer M, Evans RG, Hertzman C. Avalanche or glacier? Health care and the demographic rhetoric. 1995, webserver.ciar.ca/web/publist.nsf/PHP/C46194C39084747F8525637F004AF4EA.
4. Grundy EMD. The population aged 60 and over. *Population Trends* 1996, 84:14–20.
5. McGrail K, Green B, Barer ML, Evans RG, Hertzman C, Normand C. Age, costs of acute and long term care and proximity to death: Evidence for 1987/88 and 1994/95 in British Columbia. *Age Ageing* 2000, 29:249–253.
6. Office for National Statistics. http://www.gad.gov.uk/News/Documents/2004-based_national_population_projections.pdf. 2005.
7. GAD population projections 1994–2064 (1994 based). Population projection by sex and age for Great Britain prepared by the government actuary in consultation with the registrars general. London: Government Actuary Department, 1996.
8. Dunnell K. Are we healthier? *Population Trends* 1995, 82:12–18.
9. http://www.statistics.gov.uk/census2001/census2001.asp.
10. Wordsworth S, Donaldson C, Scott A. Can we afford the NHS? London: Institute for Public Policy Research, 1996.
11. Mendelson DN, Schwartz WB. The effects of aging and population growth on health care expenditure health care costs. *Health Affairs* 1993, 129(1): 119–125.
12. Seshamani M, Gray A. Ageing and health-care expenditure: The red herring argument revisited. *Health Economics* 2004, 13(4):303–314.
13. Graham B, Normand C, Goodall Y. Proximity to death and acute health care. Utilisation in Scotland, Information and Statistics Division, NHS, Scotland, 2003. http://www.isdscotland.org/isd/files/PTD1.pdf.
14. OECD. Ageing and income: Financial resources and retirement in 9 OECD countries. Paris, OECD 2001.

chapter eleven

Methodological issues in assessing the cost-effectiveness of interventions to improve the health of older people

Damian Walker and Cristian Aedo

Contents

Methodological issues in assessing cost-effectiveness 127
Specific objectives of improving the health of older people 129
The role of economic evaluation in health policy 129
Basic elements of cost-effectiveness analysis 130
Some core methodological issues in cost-effectiveness analysis 133
      Measurement and valuation of caregivers' time 133
      Measurement and valuation of outcomes 134
Future research and policy priorities 135
Conclusions 136
References 136

Methodological issues in assessing cost-effectiveness

At the Second World Assembly on Ageing, policy initiatives were proposed to promote active and healthy lifestyles in later life [1]. Emphasis was placed, amongst other things, on adequate nutrition throughout the life course and national food policies designed to recognise older people as potentially vulnerable. The aim was to increase healthy life-years in older people and thereby decrease the number of years, as well as the proportion of time, spent in poor health. Some governments have responded to these increased demands by designing innovative programmes aimed at tackling the twin problems of food and nutrition insecurity amongst older people [2]. For example, food baskets are still popular in some parts of Latin America, and community kitchens have also been experimented with, particularly in Argentina. In Mexico City, the local government provides a universal pension transferred electronically to a plastic debit card that can be used in supermarkets. However, to date, there is a dearth of cost, effects, and cost-effectiveness data of interventions to improve the health of older people.

The United Nations Population Division has estimated great increases in the proportion and absolute size of the older population over the next fifty years [3]. Older populations are traditionally seen as intense users of health care relative to the rest of the population, and it would thus seem logical to expect a substantial concomitant increase in health care expenditure. However, Lubitz et al. [4] estimated the relation of health status at seventy years of age to life expectancy and to cumulative health care expenditures from the age of seventy until death. They found that, despite healthier older persons' greater longevity, expected cumulative health expenditures for them were similar to those for less healthy persons. They concluded that health-promotion efforts aimed at persons under sixty-five years of age may improve the health and longevity of older people without increasing health expenditures.

The issues addressed in general health services research (e.g., optimal treatment, access to care, and the organisation of care) need to be addressed specifically with respect to the health needs of older people. Health services research is uniquely able to address the multiple factors that exert an impact upon health outcomes in later life, such as comorbidity; patient beliefs, values, and preferences; social support; and multiple sites and settings of care, as well as finance and policy factors. Health services research is multidisciplinary and conducted collaboratively by clinicians, nurses, nutritionists, and social scientists. Distinctive features of this research are its patient-centred focus and emphasis on studies related to maximising function and health-related quality of life. The 'basic sciences' of health services research are essential to this endeavour: outcomes and effectiveness research, health status measurement, economic evaluation, and quality measurement and improvement [5].

This chapter focuses on one of the 'basic sciences' of health service research—economic evaluation—and, specifically, *cost-effectiveness analysis* (CEA). The next section sets out some of the specific objectives of interventions to improve the health of older people. The following sections examine the scope of conventional forms of economic evaluation in health policy, and describe the basic elements of CEA. Thereafter, there is a description of two core methodological issues in the CEA of interventions to improve the health of older people: the measurement and valuation of caregivers' time, and the measurement and valuation of outcomes. Finally, a selection of furture research and policy priorities are listed followed by some brief conclusions.

Specific objectives of improving the health of older people

In evaluating interventions to improve the health of older people, an important initial step is the identification of their objectives. Economic evaluation, if it is to be policy relevant, needs to be matched to the actual objectives of the programmes. This section outlines the potential objectives of interventions in older people, recognising that these will vary across settings:

- *Health gain*: Examples include lives saved, years of life gained, etc. Intermediate health measures such as clinic attendance may be seen as useful tracers for change in health status, particularly given the methodological difficulties associated with measuring and attributing change in health status to an intervention.
- *Individual nonhealth benefits*: There are likely to be a number of nonhealth benefits to individuals, such as the process of care and the information resulting from these interventions.
- *Social nonhealth benefits*: This relates to changes in the wider community resulting from the programmes (e.g., community empowerment, and economic benefits such as employment and production gains). In practice some of these outcomes may have positive or negative values.

It is evident from this brief list that the objectives of such programmes do not neatly fit into unidimensional measures of health that tend to be used in cost-effectiveness studies. The next section examines in more detail the scope of such analyses.

The role of economic evaluation in health policy

The desire to implement evidence-based policy decisions has arisen as limited health care budgets have emphasised the need for providers to use resources effectively *and* efficiently. Consequently, economic evaluation has acquired greater prominence amongst decision-makers as there is a need to know which interventions represent 'value for money'.

The methods and tools of economic evaluation are rooted in the fundamental problem by which economists characterise decision-making: making choices between alternatives in the context of scarce resources. Within the scope of international and national public health, these choices are often framed in the debate as to which interventions should have priority. Economic evaluation compares the costs *and* outcomes of *at least two* alternative programmes, one of which may be 'doing nothing', although most usually is current practice [6]. There exist several types of economic evaluation, which differ in the way that outcomes or consequences are measured. They are cost-minimisation analysis, CEA, cost-utility analysis, and cost-benefit analysis.

In *cost-minimisation analysis*, two or more interventions that have identical outcomes (e.g., equal reduction in incidence of pneumonia) are assessed to see which provides the cheapest way of delivering the same outcome. CEA measures the outcome of approaches in terms of 'natural units' (e.g., for interventions in older people, this could be the number of falls prevented). *Cost-utility analysis* uses measures of utility, which reflect people's preferences, to assess outcomes. The outcomes are therefore expressed in terms of measures such as quality-adjusted life-years (QALYs) or disability-adjusted life-years (DALYs). In practice, there has been a blurring of the distinction between CEA and cost-utility analysis, with the latter seen as an extension of the former. Therefore, in this chapter, as elsewhere, the term CEA refers to both types of analysis. Finally, *cost-benefit analysis* expresses health outcomes (e.g., the number of lives saved) in terms of monetary units. The requirement of measuring outcomes in monetary units limits the use of this type of analysis in health policy.

Basic elements of cost-effectiveness analysis

The basic elements of CEA are the choice of perspective, what to include in the numerator, what to include in the denominator, how to interpret the result of CEAs, and sensitivity analysis.

The *perspective*, or *viewpoint*, relates to the scope of the evaluation. For example, analysts may adopt a narrow health care provider perspective, in which costs borne by the health care provider in question, usually the government, are captured, but those borne by the consumers of the service are excluded (e.g., the costs of accessing the service). Thus, a broader analysis may seek to collect these patient costs and would estimate costs, whoever bears them.

The costs of the intervention, borne by the provider and consumer, are sometimes supplemented by the costs of treating the disease the intervention aims to avoid; thus, treatment costs saved, or cost offsets, can be estimated. With respect to interventions in older people, treatment costs associated with pneumonia, for example, may result from outpatient visits and/or hospitalisation, other caregiver direct costs (e.g., travel), and productivity losses for caregivers. The *numerator* of the incremental cost-effectiveness ratio is thus the sum of all costs associated with delivering the service.

The *denominator* in the incremental cost-effectiveness ratio can vary. For example, process outcome measures, such as the number of older people diagnosed and treated, can be useful in order to identify the most efficient delivery system (fixed-site delivery or delivery via outreach teams). Intermediate outcome measures can be useful because they can reveal the difference between older people being effectively and ineffectively treated. In the context of interventions for older people, disease-specific outcome measures include cases of pneumonia prevented and/or treated. Examples of final outcome measures are deaths prevented and DALYs averted, which is also an example of a generic outcome measure because it enables comparisons across all types of health conditions.

The *result* of a CEA is the ratio of costs and outcomes, which represents the incremental cost per outcome of a particular alternative. It gives an idea of the relative magnitude of the cost per outcome of the alternatives. (For example, is the difference hundreds or thousands of dollars?) CEA makes the comparisons between alternatives explicit and transparent and, as such, facilitates priority-setting and hence resource allocation.

Finally, *sensitivity analysis* allows analysts to explore the impact of uncertainty on their findings. It is an important part of any economic evaluation, and a lack of analysis is evidence of a poor quality study. Sensitivity analysis helps the analyst evaluate the reliability of conclusions for the context of the evaluation and can also facilitate consideration of the generalisability of results to other settings.

An example of the methods being used in an applied CEA of a nutrition programme for older people in Chile is described next.

Cost-effectiveness analysis of a nutrition programme for older people in Chile

Chile is currently undergoing a period of rapid demographic transition that has led to an increase in the proportion of older people in the population. Many older people in Chile are socially and nutritionally vulnerable, and this has placed great demands on a national health care system with limited human resources and budget. To promote healthy ageing, the government of Chile has initiated a programme of nutritional supplementation (micronutrients and a modest amount of energy) that may have considerable positive benefits for the health and function of older people.

The overall aim of the Programme for Complementary Food in Older People (*Programa de Alimentación Complementaria para el Adulto Mayor*—PACAM) is to contribute to improvements in health and quality of life amongst older people in Chile. In order to be eligible for the programme, individuals must be registered at their local health centre and be seventy years of age or older. There are two components of PACAM: One is a powdered food called Golden Years (*Años Dorados*), which is composed of a cereal and legume mix fortified with vitamins and minerals; the other, called *Bebida Láctea*, is a similarly fortified low-lactose powdered milk. Every beneficiary is entitled to collect a 1 kg sachet of each product from his or her local health post, health centre, or hospital each month. Other elements of PACAM are monthly nutritional status assessments and nutritional and health counselling. Chile's approach to nutrition and health care has been criticised as being too expensive for most low- and middle-income countries, and therefore there is interest in evaluating the cost effectiveness of PACAM. To this end, we present a summary of methods being applied in an ongoing Wellcome Trust funded project [ISRCTN48153354], which should be of equal use for the economic evaluation of similar nutrition programmes.

Information on the types, quantities, and prices of the different 'ingredients' required to deliver PACAM is being estimated by conducting surveys and reviewing expenditure and budget records. Given that the major setup costs of the national primary health infrastructure, through which PACAM is delivered, are already covered, the additional cost of implementing PACAM corresponds to the incremental cost associated with the distribution of the two nutritional supplements and the associated staff time. Indeed, because sufficient staff time may already exist such that additional staff time is not required, we are recording how time is currently spent through time-and-motion studies. Exit interviews are being conducted to ascertain the costs of accessing the programme, focussing on the cost of transportation and the time spent accessing the programme (travel and waiting) for beneficiaries and accompanying persons. We are exploring whether lost earnings are reported.

Because the programme may result in averted cases of disease and/or additional use of health services, analysis of utilisation rates is ongoing to measure changes, and we are identifying the unit costs associated with the services averted or provided. In order to estimate the costs of these services at the individual level, we are using case-based sampling, in which, for example, individuals who have experienced episodes of pneumonia are being identified, contacted, and visited at their homes, in order to estimate the costs borne by them and any caregivers.

Based on these data, and in conjunction with the results of a controlled cluster-randomised trial, we will determine the incremental cost-effectiveness of PACAM.

It should be noted that incremental cost analyses only account for the major 'new' inputs that are required. In contrast, a full cost analysis estimates the costs of all resources employed in running a programme, including basic infrastructure. Therefore, an incremental analysis may underestimate costs of a general administrative nature borne by the provider; it is also more difficult to generalise from incremental cost analyses because it is often unclear to what extent the existing services and infrastructure are similar or not between settings. Therefore, we will perform sensitivity analysis to assess the robustness of the findings to changes in key economic and epidemiological parameters. This approach will also facilitate discussions about the generalisability of the results.

Some core methodological issues in cost-effectiveness analysis

This section addresses two issues: measurement and valuation of caregivers' time and measurement and valuation of outcomes.

Measurement and valuation of caregivers' time

Caregiving is usually characterised as formal or informal, although the distinction between the two can at times be artificial [7]. *Formal care* or support generally comes from paid professionals and public and private services organised specifically to provide a service such as home nursing, home help, or counselling. Some services, such as meals-on-wheels programmes for house-bound older people, are formally organised but often delivered partly by volunteers, making these programmes a combination of formal and informal support. *Informal care* is care provided by relatives, friends, and neighbours to older people and their families. Much informal care is provided by other older people, and is instrumental (such as help with cooking, cleaning, and shopping), personal (help with eating or toileting), and emotional (personal visits and communication). Such care is extremely important but difficult to quantify because many activities may not be recognised by the giver or receiver as 'support' or 'care'. Family members are the major providers of informal support: daughters and daughters-in-law are often the primary caregivers. Today, however, increasing joint survivorship at older ages means that the spouse (usually the wife) rather than an adult daughter often is the primary informal caregiver.

Although informal care is nominally 'free', in principle it has an economic cost because it is a resource that has alternative, valuable uses. The cost of such labour thus ideally should be based on a 'shadow price'* reflecting prevailing wage rates. The argument for such valuations is to enhance the generalisability to other, perhaps more typical, settings where such labour may need to be remunerated.

However, the difficulty in employing conventional economic approaches can be illustrated in how they deal with the issue of caregiver time, which as described earlier, can be a major factor in many programmes dealing with older people. Conventional forms of economic evaluation tend to treat volunteer and paid labour interchangeably. The assumption is that in using a shadow price for informal care based on market wage rates, one can generalise the findings to settings where informal carers are not available and

---

* A shadow price reflects the true social value of a resource.

consequently workers need to be paid. The problem, however, is that the presence and willingness of carers is often specific to the type of community in question and 'volunteerism' may be tied in with other institutional characteristics such as social capital and trust. A community that produces a supply of individuals willing to volunteer tends to be significantly different from one that does not. The features that define it as a qualitatively different input into health care from other forms of labour are the specific institutional characteristics, such as volunteerism, that it harnesses.

Quite aside from the issues of measuring and valuing caregivers' time, there is general agreement amongst researchers that the declining birth rates that accompany population ageing in many developing countries may result in fewer future caregivers for older people [8,9]. Whilst currently, in most countries, the trend of having fewer children poses greater insecurity for older people in terms of care and economic well-being, few attempts have been made to assess the impact of this decreasing fertility on family care for older people, although there are indications that it varies amongst countries [10]. It should, however, be recognised that whilst many older people receive financial and other support from adult children, support often is reciprocal. In countries with well-established pension programmes, many older adults give support and care to their children and grandchildren. Older people in less developed countries are less likely to provide financial help to younger people, but often contribute significantly to family well-being in many ways, ranging from socialisation to housekeeping to child care [7].

The implication here is that conventional forms of economic evaluation may miss important variables such as these that, in turn, contribute to the perceived value or benefit derived from such programmes. The following section examines further the failure of conventional forms of economic evaluation to capture these broader concepts of outcomes.

Measurement and valuation of outcomes

Estimating the outcomes from interventions entails deriving some measure of health gain (e.g., life-years saved) or an intermediate measure reflecting change in health risk (e.g., improved attendance at clinics). The usual difficulties, particularly in relation to detecting health gain attributable to the programmes, include inevitable time lags and controlling for confounders. These problems of attribution, however, are general to all forms of evaluation and thus will not be addressed further in this chapter.

The economic evaluations that have been undertaken to date tend largely to be conventional cost-effectiveness studies and thus based on narrowly defined endpoints (e.g., patients treated, falls avoided, cases of pneumonia averted). The value of such measures is that they provide decision-makers with explicit bases for comparing programme alternatives in terms of inputs and outputs. However, key elements of the programme can be missed through this reductionist perspective.

Examples of wider benefits that may result from interventions to improve the health of older people that are unlikely to be captured in CEA are the value attached by older people to the process of receiving such services—for example, a number of studies have shown that in low- and middle-income countries, frail older people are less respected and less valued than their healthier counterparts [11,12]—and, as alluded to earlier, institutional change. Institutions, in this sense, are defined as the patterns of behaviour that determine how individuals, groups, and organisations interact with one another [13] and may be informal (e.g., various norms of behaviour) or formal (legislation, government policy, regulations).

Institutions are relevant to programmes for older people since they are defined by specific relationships—in particular, those they establish between providers and clients (and the wider community). The development of such relationships, to some extent, alters the nature of the community. For example, they may increase the level of trust in health services and individuals' willingness to use such services; in turn, this may influence the effectiveness of future programmes. There has been recent literature [14] examining more holistic approaches to carrying out economic evaluation using institutionalist methods to account for some of these broader issues, although these themes have generally not been well recognised in economic evaluation.

Future research and policy priorities

Important gaps remain in our knowledge regarding the cost-effectiveness of interventions to improve the health of older people. Although rates of institutionalisation remain very low in most low- and middle-income countries (e.g., only 0.1% of older South Africans reside in old-age homes [15]), information is needed on how to prevent institutionalisation in a cost-effective manner and, similarly, on cost-effective models of community-based long-term care. Because long-term care creates a large burden on the family, research is needed on improving the effectiveness and cost-effectiveness of informal care, as well as relieving caregiver burden. Improvements are also needed in health status measures, especially measures adapted for the cognitively impaired and health-related quality of life (HRQOL) measures. For example, does an ageing population have implications for assessments of patient-focused health status (including patient-reported outcomes) and HRQOL?

We require reliable and valid measures for application to older population groups that can also be used within the context and for the purpose of economic evaluation. Do existing measures inherently bias cost-effectiveness results against the particular group of older people (due to older patients being less likely to benefit for long periods of time from an intervention compared to younger age groups)? Does the QALY adequately represent the health gains experienced by older people? For example, Donaldson and colleagues [16] described QALYs as being inappropriate for evaluating long-term care for older people due to insensitivity to changes in health status within this context.

Research is ongoing regarding the issues of age-weighted QALYs, where proponents of age-weighting agree that QALYs rank health care programmes correctly in terms of efficient production of health outcomes, but argue that QALYs fail to reflect public preferences for resource allocation across age groups [17–19]. However, Johri and colleagues [20] have recently argued that '…QALYs serve as a common measure of health benefits for all intervention types, age-weighting of QALYs is premature'.

Conclusions

Unprecedented changes in the demographic characteristics of countries worldwide mean that all are confronted by the challenge of preparing to meet the demands of an ageing society. In the face of current demographic trends, increasing health care costs, and concerns about the quality of health care, the financing and delivery of care for older people is a critical health care policy challenge. A focused research effort to determine how health care systems can most cost-effectively prevent disability, reduce functional decline, and extend active life expectancy in older people would provide decision-makers with the information needed to accelerate the decline in age-specific disability rates and to allocate limited resources efficiently.

This chapter has examined programmes for older people and the importance of the institutional context in defining their value or benefit. Conventional approaches to economic evaluation, particularly cost-effectiveness, tend not to capture the institutional features of such programmes. The development of a more holistic, institutionalist approach offers a potentially useful framework for evaluating such programmes.

References

1. WHO, *Active Ageing: A Policy Framework*, World Health Organisation, Geneva, 2002.
2. Dangour, A.D. et al., Chile's national nutritional supplementation program for older people: Lessons learned, *Food Nutr. Bull.*, 26, 190–197, 2005.
3. United Nations, *World Population Prospects, the 2000 Revision, Volume 1: Comprehensive Tables*. New York, United Nations, 2001.
4. Lubitz, J. et al., Health, life expectancy, and health care spending among the elderly, *N. Engl. J. Med.*, 349, 1048–1055, 2003.
5. Bierman, A. and Spector, W., Improving the health and health care of older Americans: A report of the AHRQ Task Force on Aging. Agency for Healthcare Research and Quality. Rockville, MD, 2001.
6. Drummond M. et al., *Methods for the Economic Evaluation of Health Care Programmes*, 2nd ed., Oxford University Press, Oxford, 1997.
7. Kinsella, K. and Phillips, D.R., Global aging: The challenge of success, *Population Bull.*, 60, 1–42, 2005.

8. Kendig, H., Hashimoto, A., and Coppard, L., Family support to the elderly in international perspective. In: *Family Support for the Elderly: The International Experience*, ed. Kendig, H., Hashimoto, A., and Coppard, L. Oxford, Oxford University Press, 1992.

9. Kinsella, K., *Aging in the Third World*, U.S. Bureau of the Census, Washington, D.C., 1988.

10. Levkoff, S.E., MacArthur, I.W., and Bucknall, J., Elderly mental health in the developing world, *Soc. Sci. Med.*, 41, 983–1003, 1995.

11. Glascock, A.P. and Fineman, S.L., Social asset or social burden: Treatment of the aged in nonindustrial societies. In: *Ageing, Culture and Health*, ed. Fry, C.L. J.F. Bergin Publishers, New York, 1981.

12. Guillette, E.A., Change and continuity for older Tswana, *J. Cross-Cult. Gerontol.* 5, 191–204, 1990.

13. North, D.C., Institutions and economic theory, *Am. Economist*, 36(1):3–6, 1992.

14. Jan, S., A holistic approach to the economic evaluation of health programs using institutionalist methodology, *Soc. Sci. Med.*, 47, 1565–1572, 1998.

15. Charlton, K.E. and Rose, D., Nutrition among older adults in Africa: The situation at the beginning of the millennium, *J. Nutr.*, 131, S2424–S2428, 2001.

16. Donaldson, C. et al., Should QALY's be programme specific? *J. Health Economics*, 7:239–257, 1988.

17. Nord, E. et al. The significance of age and duration of effect in social evaluation of health care, *Health Care Anal.*, 4, 103–111, 1996.

18. Tsuchiya, A., Dolan, P., and Shaw, R., Measuring people's preferences regarding ageism in health: Some methodological issues and some fresh evidence, *Soc. Sci. Med.*, 57, 687—696, 2003.

19. Williams, A., Intergenerational equity: An exploration of the 'fair innings' argument, *Health Econ.*, 6, 117–132, 1997.

20. Johri, M. et al., The importance of age in allocating health care resources: Does intervention-type matter? *Health Econ.*, 14, 669–678, 2005.

chapter twelve

Minimum income for healthy living: older people in England, 2005–2006

Jerry Morris, Alan D. Dangour, Christopher Deeming, Astrid E. Fletcher, and Paul Wilkinson

Contents

Introduction 140
Study population 140
Methods 141
Results 141
    Diet and nutrition 141
    Physical activity, anti-ageing, autonomy 142
    Housing 144
    Health care 146
    Psychosocial relations, social inclusion, active minds 147
    Hygiene: personal care and the home 147
    Getting about 148
    Other costs of healthy social living 149
    Contingencies and inefficiencies 149
    Exclusions and variations 149
Conclusions 150
Acknowledgments 151
References 151

Introduction

The loss of health, well-being, and independence as a result of inadequate income amongst older people in the United Kingdom has been extensively reviewed [1]. The House of Commons Select Committee on Social Security recommended that a minimum income standard be established for all pensioners in the United Kingdom, but it made no explicit reference to health [2]. The basic state pension (April 2006) is £84.25 a week for a single person and £134.75 for a couple. The pension credit guarantee (PCG) from April 2006 entitles pensioners aged sixty and over, after means-testing, to a weekly income at least £114.05 for single persons and £174.05 for a couple, plus winter fuel payments [3]. The latest figures show that circa 2.7 million people in Britain today receive the PCG [4]. An important question—the focus of this chapter—is the extent to which the existing benefits to which older people are entitled fall short of a minimum personal income required for healthy living (MIHL).

Whilst recognising that older people vary in their levels of health, behaviour, and social preferences, in this chapter we seek to define the requirements on average for healthy living for people aged sixty-five years or older without significant defined disability, residing in the community, and determine their realistic minimum personal expenses, as we have previously attempted for a younger age group [5].

Study population

We define our study population as those living independently (i.e., in non-assisted housing), aged sixty-five years or older and retired from paid employment. Table 12.1 provides a breakdown of this population of circa eight million in England. The proportion of people in the United Kingdom aged eighty-five years or older increased from 0.7% in 1961 to 1.9% in 2002 and is projected to rise to 3.8% of the total population in 2031. The great majority of people aged sixty-five years or older are living independently in the community (97% of men and 94% of women); however, the decline of

Table 12.1 Population Estimates for England by Age and Gender (%)

	Age groups (years)		
	65–74	75–84	85 plus
Men[a]	3.9	2.2	0.5
Women[b]	4.4	3.4	1.4
Totals	8.3	5.6	1.9

[a] Number: 3,388,200.

[b] Number: 4,558,700.

Source: National Statistics Census, London: Office for National Statistics, 2004.

independent living with age is strong, declining from 98.9% of women aged sixty-five to seventy-four years to 77.1% at eighty-five years or older. Our main focus is an MIHL for older people with no significant defined disability living in private households. This covers around 60% of the elderly population in England according to data from the Health Surveys for England.

Methods

We first derived a specification for the defined needs for healthy living in everyday terms. To do this, we drew on our expertise in each of the areas of assessment, assembling statements from international and national expert review committees, peer-reviewed topic reviews, the results of randomised controlled trials, and substantial personal observation that we judged to reflect the prevailing view of the scientific community on current best evidence. Such detailed objective evidence was occasionally lacking or not directly relevant, so we drafted pragmatic assessments that we considered would have the support of the informed health community.

We estimated realistic minimum personal costs required to meet these health needs currently in England, using two methods. For most items we made enquiries into representative prices from familiar low cost retailers/ suppliers. Where we were unable to define a cost in this way we resorted to data from national surveys on the average actual weekly expenditure by households in the lowest 40% of incomes where the head of household was aged sixty-five years or older. Many such costs were derived from the national Expenditure and Food Surveys, 2002–2004 [6]. Table 12.2 provides further information on the source of data used in the current study.

Results

Diet and nutrition

The importance of good nutrition for the maintenance of health and function in older people is well recognised [7]. The current healthy diet was constructed using an international expert report on good nutrition for older people [7] and U.K. guidance for healthy eating [8–10].

Three stages were employed in designing the diet. First, the level of daily energy intake was calculated based on the predicted requirement for moderately active men and women aged seventy-five to eighty-four in the United Kingdom [11,12]. Second, an indicative diet was constructed that, over the course of seven days, met the macro- and micronutrient requirements of older people (Table 12.3) [7,8,13]. Older people absorb vitamin B_{12} from their food poorly or not at all, and vitamin B_{12} (2.5 µg/day) was therefore provided in easily absorbed crystalline form via a daily dietary supplement [7]. Salt intake was higher than recommended but would be reduced by up to 37% with the provision of low-salt bread and breakfast cereal. Third, the diet was designed to meet internationally accepted food-based dietary guidelines [7].

Table 12.2 Main Sources of Data Used in Calculation of Minimum Income for Healthy Living in Older People

	Item	Data sources
Diet/ nutrition	Food and drink costs	*De novo* survey using online shopping facility
Physical activity	Equipment, charges	Direct costing; local shops, local authorities
Housing	Insurance, water services	National Expenditure and Food Survey (EFS)
	Fuel costs	Standardized estimates, English House Condition Survey (EHCS)
	Maintenance and breakdown	Published contract prices; required repair costs, EHCS; Expenditure and Food Survey
Health care	Dental care	Dental Practice Board
	Spectacles/lenses	Department of Health
Psychosocial relations	Memberships, subscriptions, and miscellaneous items	Direct costing
Getting about	Buses, taxis, cycles, etc.	Direct costing

Half of the diet was priced at a leading lower price U.K. supermarket, and store-label, low-cost products were selected where available; the other half was priced at customarily more expensive local shops [5]. We then allowed a further 10% for wastage [14]. The cost of the healthy diet is £32.30 per week for moderately active single men and women and £63.70 per week for a moderately active couple.

Physical activity, anti-ageing, autonomy

Modern research has established the needs for physical activity across the life span. The benefits—physical (e.g., mobility essential for active ageing), psychological, and social—apply to men and women alike and the potential for benefit is there at all ages, including those over sixty-five years.

Currently, most of the older population in the United Kingdom does not take enough exercise [15]. Extensive evidence [15–19] on the multiple health benefits of physical activity in older age led us to emphasise the importance of activity for health in daily living. The benefits of regular physical activity include: countering ageing processes (e.g., partially making good the loss of muscle mass and strength and heart-lung capacity, which decline by about 1% a year from the forties); weight regulation; improvement of lipid profile and blood pressure, and reduction of cardiovascular and diabetes risks; and generally in improving quality of independent daily living by improving mobility and other physical capabilities, possibly also mental capabilities, often in the presence of long-term disabilities.

Table 12.3 Average Daily Nutrient Composition of Our 'Healthy Diet' Compared to International[a] and National[b] Recommendations and Safe Upper Levels of Intake[c]

	Moderately active men	Moderately active women	WHO/ TUFTS[a]	DoH[b]	SUL[c]
Energy (kcal)	2439.0	2085.0	2059–2648	2100	
Protein (g)	105.8	90.3	65.6–80.2	53.3	
Englyst fibre (g)	27.6	24.1			
Sodium (mg)[d]	3330.0	2760.0		1600	
Potassium (mg)	4706.0	4221.0		3500	
Calcium (mg)	1052.0	904.0	800–1200	700	
Magnesium (mg)	505.0	438.0	225–280	300	
Phosphorus (mg)	1931.0	1667.0		550	
Iron (mg)	23.6	20.3	10	8.7	
Copper (mg)	2.0	1.7	1.3–1.5	1.2	10.0
Zinc (mg)	13.2	11.3	7	9.5	25.0
Selenium (µg)	112.0	85.0	50–70	75	450.0
Iodine (µg)	137.0	130.0		140	
Vitamin A (µg) RE	996.0	975.0	600–700	700	
Vitamin C (mg)	193.0	190.0	60–100	40	
Vitamin D (µg)	11.6	9.8	10.0–15.0	10	
Vitamin E (mg)	6.5	6.1	4.3–17.2	4	34.5
Thiamin (mg)	2.4	2.1		0.9	
Riboflavin (mg)	2.4	2.1	1.3	1.3	
Niacin equivalents (mg)	56.0	47.3		16	
Vitamin B6 (mg)	3.3	2.9		1.4	10.0
Vitamin B12 (µg)	12.1[e]	9.3[e]	2.5[f]	1.5	
Total folate (µg)	454.0	406.0	400	200	
Pantothenic acid (mg)	5.9	5.4		3.0–7.0	
Biotin (µg)	50.3	46.6		10–200	
Alcohol (g)	11.9	11.9			
Percentage of energy from					
Protein %	17.3	17.4			
Total fat %	29.5	29.4	30	33	
Saturates %	8.5	8.2	8	10	
Monounsaturates %	11.0	11.1			
Polyunsaturates %	6.8	6.9			
Carbohydrate %	49.3	49.1		47	
Sugars %	23.7	23.8			
Starch %	25.7	25.3			
Alcohol %	3.9	4.0			

[a] WHO/TUFTS, Keep fit for life: Meeting the nutritional needs of older persons. Geneva: World Health Organisation, 2002.

[b] Department of Health. The nutrition of elderly people: Report of the working group on the nutrition of elderly people of the Committee on Medical Aspects of Food Policy, 1992.

[c] Expert Group on Vitamins and Minerals. Safe upper levels of vitamins and minerals. London: Food Standards Agency; 2003.

[d] The sodium intake is higher than recommended and would be reduced by up to 37% with the provision of low-salt (but high-cost) bread and breakfast cereal.

[e] Not including intake from B12 supplement.

[f] As supplement.

We focussed on three areas: (1) dynamic aerobic exercise, such as walking and swimming for heart and lung and general wellbeing; (2) physical activity for strengthening the muscles (i.e., activity against some resistance for building muscle mass and strength); and (3) activities such as bending and stretching that help foster mobility, flexibility, balance, and stability.

We aimed to promote habitual, appropriate, and enjoyable exercise amongst older people that should be absorbed into the daily routine. In our estimates of the cost of such exercise, we allowed for a weekly group exercise session or solo swim at a local authority venue (weekly cost £1.50 for a single person, £3.00 for a couple) and also provided basic clothing expenses needed for a regular regimen of walking, swimming, and similar exercise (totalling £0.60/week for a single person, £1.10/week for a couple for inexpensive swimming kit, etc.). The costs of extra calories and laundry were covered under other appropriate headings.

Housing

Housing has been a central concern of public health from its modern beginnings. There is broad recognition that decent housing is important for many aspects of healthy living [20], particularly in the older population, which spends much of its time at home and indoors. A healthy home therefore needs to have sound structure, to be free of hazards, to provide adequate facilities for sleeping, personal hygiene, preparation and storage of food, to provide an environment for comfortable relaxation, and to offer facilities for privacy, and for communication and social exchange with friends, family, and others.

We were unable to translate many of these requirements into specific costs. We used average housing expenditure for insurance and water service charges (for which rebates cannot normally be claimed), but did not include council tax, rent, and mortgage payments, the costs of which are claimable after further means-testing by those on low income (and excluded these also in our figures of the PCG). To these costs, we added two further items that have specific bearing on health in older people: fuel costs and maintenance and repair costs.

Epidemiological evidence suggests that mortality in people aged sixty-five years or more is 20 to 30% greater in winter than in other months [21,22]. Much of this winter excess is attributable to cold [23]. Although some of the cold-related risk may arise through short-term excursions outdoors [24], there is evidence that poor housing, in particular inadequate home heating, increases vulnerability to winter death [21,25]. Fuel costs, including those needed to heat the home to the minimum heating standard, were obtained from the 2001 English House Conditions Survey [26]. We took these adequate standardised fuel costs for dwellings of people in the lowest quartile of the income distribution and translated them to a weekly average for the year as a whole.

Good maintenance and repair of a dwelling is important for safety. Older people in particular are at risk of falls, including falls on the level, down stairs, and in bath accidents, and they are at risk from fires and other hazards, most of which occur in the home [27,28]. There are also safety issues arising from poor maintenance of gas boilers and other heating appliances because of the potential for incomplete combustion of fuel and the consequent risk of carbon monoxide release [29]. It is important too that boilers are not at risk of failure during the critical periods of coldest weather. More than most other groups, the elderly are often concerned with security, for which good maintenance of doors and windows is necessary. We therefore consider costs for maintenance and repair as core elements of our minimum income estimates and include a maintenance contract covering four main areas: central heating, other gas appliances, the electrical system, and plumbing and drains. We based our figures on the contract offered by British Gas, which is probably the best known and competitive, if not necessarily the cheapest, available.

To these we have added figures from the 2002–2004 Expenditure and Food Surveys to reflect the actual spending of households on dwelling and other repairs not included elsewhere in this report. We reasoned that this (inadequate) level of expenditure, which reflects 'average' practice amongst low-income households, should be added to the annualised cost for making a dwelling fit in order to achieve the required total for maintenance and repair.

Finally, we added a basic cost to make the dwelling fit for habitation. Data from the 2001 English House Conditions Survey (EHCS) [26] indicate that many dwellings are not kept in good repair and require significant expenditure to make them fit for habitation (e.g., to treat dampness, repair roofs). This suggests that many people spend less on repairs than necessary, so, to estimate requisite costs, we included a combination of EHCS estimates of the 'cost to make a fit for habitation' and actual household expenditure on maintenance and repairs. As detailed in Table 12.4, the weekly total costs summed to £36.55 for a single person sixty-five years or older and £39.48 for a couple.

Table 12.4 Housing Costs, per Week

	Cost (pounds)	
	Single	Couple
Water supply and miscellaneous services relating to the dwelling	6.21	6.26
Fuel costs for heating and cooking	13.75	13.75
Insurance (dwelling, structural, and contents)	2.65	3.54
Maintenance, breakdown and repairs of heating system, etc.	6.97	6.97
Basic repair costs to make dwelling fit for habitation	3.51	3.51
Repairs and maintenance of dwelling fabric	3.46	5.45
Total	36.55	39.48

Health care

All our population aged sixty-five or older are entitled without cost to GP and NHS hospital services. The following services are also offered without cost to these people:

- NHS prescriptions are provided.
- NHS sight tests are provided.
- Hearing aids: Reduced hearing is increasingly common as age advances, but surveys suggest that nearly half of those with reduced hearing do not have a hearing aid [30]. Hearing aids, including modern digital aids, are free to all on the NHS [31].
- Flu vaccination for people is provided.
- Antipneumococcal vaccination: This is currently offered free at age seventy-five or older and, from 2005 to 2006, to all aged sixty-five or older. It is not needed each year and for most it is a one-off vaccination [32].
- Patients aged seventy-five years and over may request a consultation for a health check by their GP if they have not had a consultation within the previous twelve months [33].

However, we also included three specific items. The first of these is ophthalmic services. Whilst NHS sight tests (visual acuity, general eye check, intraocular pressure), recommended at biennial (under age seventy) or annual frequency [34], are free, lenses and frames (which are needed by almost everyone in this age group) are not. Their costs were estimated from the average weekly spending on eye care of people sixty-five years or older in the lowest 40% of the income distribution: £0.80 for a single person or £1.60 for a couple. State help is provided for these costs for those receiving PCG or with a partial exemption certificate.

The second additional item is dental care. Dental services are currently under review [35], but at present, old age itself does not give exemption from NHS dental charges in England. Because we were unable to define from first principles the necessary expenditure that may be entailed, we again took figures for the (probably inadequate) actual expenditure for NHS patients aged sixty-five to seventy-four in England and Wales: £0.70 for a single person and £1.40 for a couple, per week.

Finally, over-the-counter medicines are commonly used by older people and thus were added to the allowance. Although their health benefits and appropriateness have not been well researched, we allowed these and costed them using actual expenditure data for the lowest 40% of the income distribution [36]: £0.50 for a single person or £1.00 for a couple.

The total weekly personal costs of health care are £2.00 for a single person and £4.00 for a couple.

Psychosocial relations, social inclusion, active minds

Psychosocial relations and social inclusion are critical for physical, mental, and social health in older people [37–41]. Government attaches particular importance to the avoidance of social exclusion and its significance for social cohesion and social capital as well as for personal health [42,43]. Such belonging and contributing, together with the ties of personal relationships, physical competence, and financial capability, make for personal autonomy in older age. There is also growing evidence that mental activity, social engagement, and mental stimulation during older age can slow mental decline [44,45]. However, social roles with their mutual obligations and group membership all incur money costs to the individual.

Some services that facilitate social and cultural integration and lively minds are often free at the point of use; these include public libraries, television, book clubs, art galleries, and museums. However, we allowed costs for other important resources such as newspapers, the theatre, concerts, and the occasional café meal. In the present study, we average TV costs to allow the licence for those under age seventy-five; for persons that age or older this is free in the United Kingdom. Those over age sixty-five spend three and three-quarter hours on average a day watching television, one and three-quarter hours reading [46], and two and a half hours listening to the radio [47].

We have specified minimal personal costs as a telephone, occasional gifts to grandchildren and others, modest recreational and entertainment costs, a television set (and licence for those under age seventy-five), a daily newspaper, an annual U.K. holiday, and a little money for hobbies and the like. This list, which could be varied in its detail, represents our collective judgement of the range of needs essential for maintaining reciprocal ties with relations, friends, and the wider community; social participation with all its manifold personal and public benefits; and an active mind (Table 12.5).

Hygiene: personal care and the home

Hygiene has two main functions. It serves to maintain healthy living by combating agents of infectious disease in the person and the home, and it functions socially and psychologically by promoting connections and supporting personal esteem and respect. Some limited evidence highlights the importance of washing hands with soap, which can reduce the risk of diarrhoeal infection by almost half [48] and of keeping dishcloths and clothes clean. There is also much concern today with care in food storage and preparation.

Direct evidence of the role of hygiene in maintaining the quality of older people's lives is scarce. Clearly, without a minimum level of grooming there is risk of social exclusion. Clean hair, use of soap and deodorant, clothes washed with detergent, a shaved face, and styled hair are all often expected in normal social interaction. Similarly, a house that is not tidy, with washed

Table 12.5 Pyschosocial Relations, Social Inclusion, Active
Minds, Costs per Week[a]

	Cost (pounds)	
	Single	Couple
Telephone	4.00	4.00
Stationery, stamps	0.40	0.40
Gifts to grandchildren, others	1.70	1.60
Subscriptions, social clubs, etc.	2.00	4.00
Cinema, sports, etc.	1.00	2.00
Meeting friends, entertaining	1.20	2.30
Television set and licence	1.70	1.70
Newspapers	2.40	2.40
Holidays (U.K.)	3.20	7.10
Miscellaneous, hobbies, gardening, etc.	3.90	5.60
Total	21.50	31.10

[a] We assumed that books are obtained from the public library, the
   local newspaper is free, and there is no cost for radio.

utensils, a clean bathroom, and free of wastes, will not encourage family and
friends to visit.

Minimum needs of hygiene for aesthetic and social reasons are combined
with physical health in the minimum weekly costs allowed of £4.80 for a
single person and £7.80 for a couple.

Getting about

Necessary minimal expenditure for 'getting about' is largely derived from
special analysis of data in the Department for Transport National Travel
Survey (NTS) 2000. We focus on public transport, particularly travel by bus,
but have also allowed for taxis and occasional journeys by train. On-peak
bus travel is assumed to be at concessionary rates and with an annual bus
pass. For some older people, however, particularly in rural areas, public
transport is limited, not serving the right places at the right times. NTS data
suggest taxi use to be three times greater amongst older people in rural areas.

Walking is, of course, the basic and healthy, low-cost mode of getting
about for older people. It is also an often unavoidable element in travel by
public transport. The NTS reports that nearly a third of trips by people age
sixty-five or older are made on foot. The potential of bicycle use in the United
Kingdom by younger, fit, old people has been neglected compared with
Holland and Denmark, for example, where it is popular and catered for. This
is a healthy, low-cost way of getting about and we therefore make some
allowance for it. Personal transport in the form of a car is not considered a
necessary requirement for healthy living; this is particularly so where availability and accessibility of public transport are satisfactory. Moreover, the
costs associated with owning a car have been reported to be up to 24% of

the total weekly expenditure of households in the lowest income quintile that have cars [49].

Minimum personal weekly costs of getting about based on bus, rail, taxi, and cycle costs are £3.20 for a single person and £6.30 for a couple.

Other costs of healthy social living

Inevitably, there are gaps in current scientific knowledge related to health. To fill these gaps and arrive at a realistic total assessment of healthy living costs, we therefore used family spending data from the 2002–2004 national Expenditure and Food Survey [50]. Our figures are based on the average weekly spending by those in the lowest 40% of incomes where the head of household is aged sixty-five or older. We allowed £2.70 a week for a single person (£8.00 for a couple) for clothing, footwear, and laundry, and £9.10 a week for a single person (£15.30 for a couple) for household goods and services.

Contingencies and inefficiencies

People are required to save for contingencies—for example, for breakdowns and for funeral expenses. Moreover, we cannot assume that all older people, in real life, will be able to meet MIHL with the level of efficiency that our experts used in its construction. Some will be less efficient and it may be for reasons beyond their control. For example, we constructed the basic diet using the cheapest value products of the particular low-cost chain, but these products can occasionally be out of stock and a branded equivalent is likely to be more expensive. Recognising this, other investigators have allowed for such 'inefficiencies', and in line with Beveridge's 1942 report on social security, we have allowed 6% for inefficiencies [51]. We allowed £1.40 a week for savings for a single person and for a couple.

Exclusions and variations

Expenditures for smoking, gambling, and alcoholic drink (except for modest alcohol consumption with food and the cost of one drink out every fortnight) are excluded from MIHL because they are bad for health. In addition, we have not been able to make allowance for personal preferences and choice.

The aim of our study has been to construct a single itemised MIHL for those aged sixty-five years or older, singles and couples, to compare with current U.K. government policy. During the study, we observed variations in relation to age, gender, and location, but the present study has not attempted any sensitivity analysis of costs and prices. On occasions where we found significant variation, we took pragmatic averages to achieve single costs to produce MIHL.

Table 12.6 Summary of Personal Costs: Minimum Personal Income Required for Healthy Living: MIHL. Older People without Significant Disability Living in the Community, England, April 2005

	Cost (pounds)	
	Single	Couple
Diet/nutrition	32.30	63.70
Physical activity	2.10	4.10
Housing	36.60	39.50
Health care	2.00	4.00
Psychosocial relations, social inclusion, and active minds	21.50	31.10
Hygiene	4.80	7.80
Getting about	3.20	6.30
Other costs of healthy social living	11.80	23.30
Contingencies/inefficiencies	8.40	12.30
Total April 2005	122.70	192.10
Total MIHL at April 2006 prices	126.00	200.00

Conclusions

Our aim in this study was to translate, for the first time, current best evidence of essential health needs in older people into an income requirement. We hope to stimulate debate about an area of public policy that hitherto has paid too little attention to questions of health and health inequalities. Our findings show that the current state pension in England and the official safety net, the pension credit guarantee of £114.05 for single persons and £174.05 for couples, fall below our estimated minimum personal income required for healthy living (Table 12.6). Moreover, the PCG will often also have to meet additional costs of disability which are excluded from the present study. This suggests that income is a barrier to healthy living for many older people who have no other income but the state PCG.

However, many older people may not have the knowledge, inclination, or situation to spend as we have indicated, and even though we have allowed for inefficiencies, contingencies, and wastage, our MIHL budget may yet represent a considerable challenge if minimal requirements for health are to be met. A national commitment to a minimum income for healthy living could therefore also be a powerful stimulus for national public health, education, and cultural change.

Our costing of current best evidence should be regarded as indicative rather than definitive for several reasons. First, several elements were unavoidably based on actual expenditure by low-income families rather than on need. However, these expenditure data probably fall below the level necessary for health. This is most likely the case for items without immediate necessity, such as insurance, on which those with low income may be tempted to economise. Second, we were unable to pay adequate attention to the potentially substantial variations in costs amongst individuals, sub-populations, and areas.

We also propose that the MIHL approach provides an alternative way of defining poverty that supplements the official definition in terms of 60% of current median income. We suggest the MIHL approach provides a different perspective on poverty and income standards, which hitherto have made too little reference to the growing body of knowledge on health.

Acknowledgments

This research was largely funded by a grant from Age Concern England, whose support is gratefully acknowledged. PW was supported by a Public Health Career Scientist Award (NHS Executive, CCB/BS/PIICS031). We thank numerous colleagues for comments, advice, and information.

References

1. Acheson D. *Independent Inquiry into Inequalities in Health*. London: The Stationery Office; 1998.
2. Select Committee on Social Security. Seventh report. London: House of Commons, The United Kingdom Parliament, 2000.
3. Chancellor of the Exchequer. *Opportunity for All: The Strength to Take the Long-Term Decisions for Britain*. Pre-budget report December 2004. Cm 6408. London: HM Treasury, 2004.
4. Department for Work and Pensions. *Pension Credit Quarterly Statistical Enquiry: March 2005*. London: DWP, 2005.
5. Morris JN, Donkin AJ, Wonderling D, Wilkinson P, Dowler EA. A minimum income for healthy living. *J Epidemiol Community Health* 2000, 54(12):885–889.
6. National Statistics. *Family Spending: Reports on the 2002–04 Expenditure and Food Survey*. London: The Stationary Office, 2004, 5.
7. WHO/Tufts. Keep fit for life: Meeting the nutritional needs of older persons. Geneva: World Health Organisation, 2002.
8. Department of Health. The nutrition of elderly people: Report of the working group on the nutrition of elderly people of the Committee on Medical Aspects of Food Policy, 1992.
9. Scientific Advisory Committee on Nutrition. *Salt and Health*. London: The Stationary Office, 2003.
10. Scientific Advisory Committee on Nutrition. *Advice on Fish Consumption: Benefits and Risks*. London: The Stationary Office, 2004.
11. FAO/WHO/UNU. Human energy requirements: Report of a joint FAO/WHO/UNU expert consultation. Rome: Food and Agriculture Organisation, 2004.
12. Finch S, Doyle W, Lowe C, et al. National diet and nutrition study—People aged 65 years and over. London: HMSO, 1998.
13. Expert Group on Vitamins and Minerals. Safe upper levels of vitamins and minerals. London: Food Standards Agency, 2003.
14. Department for Environment Food and Rural Affairs. *National Food Survey 2000*. London: The Stationary Office, 2001.

15. Department of Health. At least five a week: Evidence on the impact of physical activity and its relationship to health. A report from the chief medical officer. 2004.

16. Young A, Dinan S. Active in later life. In: *ABC of Sports Medicine*, ed. King, J. London: BMA, 2000, 51–56.

17. U.S. Department of Health and Human Services. Physical activity and health: A report of the surgeon general. Washington, DC: Centers for Disease Control and Prevention, National Center for Chronic Disease Prevention and Health Promotion, 1996.

18. Morris JN, Hardman AE: Walking to health. *Sports Med* 1997, 23:306–332; 324, 396.

19. Rejeski WJ, Brawley LR, Haskell WL. Physical activity: Preventing physical disablement in older adults. *Am J Prev Med* 2003, 25(3 Suppl 2).

20. BMA. Housing and health: Building for the future. 2003.

21. Wilkinson P, Landon M, Armstrong B, Stevenson S, McKee M. *Cold Comfort: The social and environmental determinants of excess winter death in England, 1986–1996*. York: Joseph Rowntree Foundation, 2001.

22. Wilkinson P, Pattenden S, Armstrong B, Fletcher A, Kovats RS, Mangtani P, McMichael AJ. Vulnerability to winter mortality in elderly people in Britain: Population-based study. *BMJ* 2004, 329(7467):647.

23. Armstrong B, Wilkinson P, Stevenson S. Identifying components of seasonal variation in mortality. *Epidemiology* 2000, 11(4):S113.

24. The Eurowinter Group. Cold exposure and winter mortality from ischaemic heart disease, cerebrovascular disease, respiratory disease, and all causes in warm and cold regions of Europe. *Lancet* 1997, 349:1341–1346.

25. Warm Front Study Group. National evaluation of the health impacts of England's home energy efficiency programme (Warm Front). Report to DEFRA. 2004.

26. Office of the Deputy Prime Minister. English House Conditions Survey. 2001.

27. Ormandy D, Battersby S, Landon M, Moore R, Wilkinson P. Statistical evidence to support the housing health and safety rating system. Vol 1—Project report. London: Office of the Deputy Prime Minister, 2003.

28. Ormandy D, Battersby S, Landon M, Moore R, Wilkinson P. Statistical evidence to support the housing health and safety rating system. Vol 2—Summary of results. London: Office of the Deputy Prime Minister, 2003.

29. IEH. Assessment on indoor air quality in the home (2): Carbon monoxide. Leicester: Institute for Environment and Health, 1998.

30. Smeeth L, Fletcher AE, Siu-Woon Ng E, Stirling S, Nunes M, Breeze E, Bulpitt CJ, Jones D, Tulloch AJ. Reduced hearing, ownership, and use of hearing aids in elderly people in the U.K.—The MRC Trial of the Assessment and Management of Older People in the Community: A cross-sectional survey. *Lancet* 2002, 359:1466–1470.

31. All about hearing aids (http://www.rnid.org.uk/html/leaflets/all_about_hearing_aids.htm).

32. Department of Health. Pneumococcal vaccine for older people (fact-sheet). London: DoH Publications, 2003.

33. Department of Health. Delivering investment in general practice: Implementing the new GMS contract. London: DH, 2003.

34. College of Optometrists. *Good Optometric Practice: Code of Ethics and Guidance for Professional Conduct*. London: College of Optometrists, 2003.

35. U.S. Department of Health and Human Services and U.S. Department of Agriculture. *Dietary Guidelines for Americans*, 2005. 6th ed. Washington, DC: Government Printing Office, 2005.

36. Boulos M, Phillipps G. Is NHS dentistry in crisis? 'Traffic light' maps of dentists' distribution in England and Wales. *Int J Health Geogr* 2004, 3:10.

37. Cassel J. The contribution of the social environment to host resistance. *Am J Epidemiol* 1976, 104:107–123.

38. Berkman LF. The relationship of social networks and social support to morbidity and mortality. In: *Social Support and Health*, ed. Syme, ST. Orlando, FL: Academic Press, 1985.

39. Berkman LF, Kawachi I (eds.). *Social Epidemiology.* Oxford, New York: Oxford University Press, 2000.

40. WHO. *Active Ageing: a policy framework. WHO*, Geneva, 2002.

41. Dalgard OS, Haheim LL. Psychosocial risk factors and mortality: A prospective study with special focus on social support, social participation, and locus of control in Norway. *J Epidemiol Community Health* 1998, 52:476–481.

42. Social Exclusion Unit. Tackling Social Exclusion: Taking stock and looking to the future: Emerging findings. The Stationary Office. 2004.

43. Szreter S, Woolcock M. Health by association? Social capital, social theory, and the political economy of public health. *Int J Epidemiol* 2004, 33(4):650–667.

44. Fratiglioni L, Paillard-Borg S, Winblad B. An active and socially integrated lifestyle in late life might protect against dementia. *Lancet Neurol* 2004, 3(6):343–353.

45. Coyle JT. Use it or lose it—Do effortful mental activities protect against dementia? *N Engl J Med* 2003, 348:2489–2490.

46. National Statistics. U.K. 2000 Time Use Survey. 2003.

47. Office for National Statistics. *Social Focus on Older People*. London: The Stationery Office, 1999.

48. Netten A, Curtis L. Unit costs of health and social care 2002. Report of the Personal Social Services Research Unit. Canterbury: University of Kent, 2002.

49. Social Exclusion Unit. Making the connections: Final report on transport and social exclusion. 2003.

50. National Statistics. *Family Food: A Report of the 2002–03 Expenditure and Food Survey.* London: The Stationary Office, 2004.

51. Beveridge W. *Social Insurance and Allied Services*. Cmd 6404. London. HMSO, 1942.

52. National Statistics. Healthy life expectancy for Great Britain and England: Annual estimates 1981 to 2001. London: Office for National Statistics, 2004.

chapter thirteen

Responding to increasing human longevity: policy, practice, and research

David Metz

Contents

Increasing longevity 155
Implications of increased longevity 156
Health 158
Functional decline 162
Conclusion 163
References 163

Increasing longevity

Human longevity has been increasing, in part as a consequence of the sorts of advances in understanding and practice discussed in this symposium. What of the future? In its most recent population projections, the United Kingdom Government Actuary's Department adopted more optimistic assumptions than previously about future improvements in mortality. Previous projections had assumed that rates of mortality improvement would gradually diminish in the long term. Thus, the 2002-based projections assumed that the historic rate of mortality improvement of 1% a year would apply for the next twenty-five years but would halve every twenty-five years thereafter. However, expectations of life at birth have continued to rise at relatively constant rates over the last twenty years for males and females, suggesting that the previous long-term assumptions have been too pessimistic. Accordingly, for the 2004-based projections, the rates of improvement are now assumed to remain constant at 1% per annum for the indefinite future [1].

The government actuary seems to be moving in the direction of those optimists amongst the demographers who predict that a baby girl born in Britain this year will, on average, live for a full century [2,3]. There are, however, demographic pessimists who view the rise in obesity, especially in the United States, as likely to bring to an end the steady increase in life expectancy of the past two centuries [4]. Another threat is infectious disease, with pandemic influenza a particular concern.

Whilst obesity and infectious disease have the potential to affect future average life expectancy, the main impact, arguably, is likely to be to increase inequalities. Readers of this chapter, for instance, are much less likely to suffer from obesity than the average person. Whilst any of us might be struck down by infectious disease, the longevity prospects for the survivors seem unlikely to be much altered. Thus, it is reasonable to suppose that, at least for large sections of the population of the United Kingdom and similar countries, increasing longevity is the future reality.

Implications of increased longevity

Increasing longevity is, of course, a triumph of human progress. But we are anxious about the consequences: about the financing of pensions, about health-care costs, and—as yet less well articulated—about economic competitiveness.

Stories about setbacks to pension prospects are frequently to be found in the newspapers nowadays. One reason is that the expectation of increasing longevity is undermining the actuarial basis of occupational pension schemes. A 'funding gap' is developing. The independent Pensions Commission, established by the U.K. government, issued its final report in November 2005 [5]. The commission identified three approaches to tackling the pension problem: raising taxes or national insurance; increasing savings; or raising the average retirement age. The government has broadly accepted the commission's proposals [6]. At the same time, the government has introduced regulations to implement a European Union directive on age discrimination in employment. This will preclude contractual retirement ages below sixty-five and allow employees to request to work on past the retirement age.

Thus, we have increasing longevity contributing to the pensions' funding gap. We also have a later start to working life as higher education becomes more prevalent. It therefore seems inevitable that we shall have to work for longer, rather than retire earlier. It is just not possible to sustain thirty years of retirement on pension entitlement built up over only thirty years of full-time work. Fortunately, the virtues of older workers are increasingly recognised by business, particularly relevant in those prosperous parts of the country where there are skills shortages (see, for instance, Population Ageing Associates [7]). The retail, financial services, and health-care sectors, which deal face to face with their customers, also appreciate the case for matching the demographic profile of their staff to that of their clients. The National Health Service, Britain's largest employer, is particularly enlightened, allowing staff to wind down to retirement by working part-time in the same post, whilst continuing to build pension entitlement, or to step down, working full-time but in a more junior role, as well as continuing to work after retirement, thus earning and taking pension [8].

The employment rate of people in Britain between age fifty and state pension age (currently sixty-five for men and sixty for women) has been rising in recent years, from 66% in 1999 to 71% in 2005 [9]. Maintaining this rising trend will only be possible if the work suits the capabilities of the worker. We recognise the development of multiple minor disabilities as we age, so there is a need to promote the health of the work force and adapt the working environment to their needs—a concept known as 'work ability' and pioneered in Finland. This involves ergonomic adaptations to the work place, training workers in new technology and training managers to manage older workers, as well as provision of occupational health services [10,11].

There are, of course, anxieties about longer working lives, particularly on the part of those involved in heavy, stressful, or unfulfilling work. Nevertheless, work, whether paid or unpaid, can foster social connectedness and social support, which are good for health in later life; moreover, older people believe in the value of productive life [12]. Therefore, it is likely that good work—that is, the right kind of work— is good for health and well-being. The challenge, then, for policy, practice, and research is to devise approaches that meet the needs of older workers and their employers. The main requirement is to eliminate any gap between the capabilities of the worker and the capabilities demanded by the job.

Longer working lives are one element of a national response to population ageing. The issue of economic vigour and competitiveness needs also to be addressed. What will it be like to live in a society in which the average age of an adult is fifty, as will be the case in Britain in the 2020s? Does this necessarily imply a loss of competitiveness vis-à-vis societies with younger populations? Here, there is a dearth of definitive evidence. But there are some interesting pointers. Individuals starting their business around the age of fifty have higher survival rates in business than do younger workers, suggesting, perhaps, that experience may be more important than enthusiasm [13].

There are also clues from studies of artistic and other kinds of creativity. Galenson [14,15] has studied the output of modern artists according to the age at which they produce their work (e.g., comparing the value of the outputs of Picasso and Cezanne), using as yardsticks the frequency with which the works of each artist are to be found in the illustrated art textbooks and prices achieved at auction. Galenson distinguishes two types of innovator. Conceptual innovators, such as Picasso, desire to communicate specific ideas and generate innovations that seem suddenly to appear; they tend to produce their best work fairly early in their careers, when they challenge accepted wisdom. Thus, Picasso produced his highest value output in his third decade. In contrast, the goals of experimental innovators—Cezanne, for instance—are ambitious but vague; they work by trial and error to produce their major contributions over an extended period of time, generally creating their most valuable work later in life as they accumulate the evidence and experience that underpins their achievements. Cezanne's most valuable work was painted in his final decade of life. Galenson has applied this kind of analysis not only to artists, but also to poets, novelists, and economists, and draws similar conclusions.

Accordingly, we need not be pessimistic about the scope for human innovation as the centre of gravity of the population increases, as the age shift moves us towards an older world. Improvements based on experience might match a shift in the wants and needs of people as the customer base ages. Perhaps interest in new material possessions might decline, to be replaced by a desire to maintain health and autonomy and a focus on self-realisation. Those who have recently retired are financially better off than previous generations of pensioners, benefiting from the buildup of occupational and personal pensions, with the rate of poverty now about the same as amongst nonpensioner groups. Notwithstanding concerns about the level of future pensions discussed earlier, many older people today have substantial purchasing power and can increasingly choose their preferred lifestyle. The most recent cohort of retirees has grown up with the 'consumer society' and is accustomed to exercising choice. Consumption by older consumers is a topic attracting growing academic and business interest [16,17].

Health

One important area of consumption for older people is health care, whether funded through taxation, insurance, or direct purchase. The prospect of further population ageing would seem to point to ever growing health-care expenditure. However, a person's need for medical expenditure over the life course is concentrated in the final year or two of life [18–20]. Thus, increasing longevity in itself would be expected to defer the timing of this late life expenditure, without having much effect on total health-care expenditure over the life course. However, health expenditure for the population is set to rise for two reasons. First, the large baby boom generation will in due course increase the numbers of those reaching the end of life. In Britain this will add an additional two million older people to those over age seventy in the 2030s, who will amount to some ten million in total. Second, demand for health care rises as people get richer and have met other, more basic needs. The proportion of GDP spent on health care has been rising in all developed countries, typically doubling over the past forty years, and currently exceeds 10% in a number of OECD countries [21]. We can expect this to continue to increase because of the value that people place on good health.

Nordhaus [22] has estimated the economic value of the increase in life expectancy over the past half century brought about by health technologies, both medical advances and public health improvements. He has compared this with the benefits from advances in nonhealth technologies—for instance, transport, communications, and computers. He concludes that, to a first approximation, the economic value of improvements in health status over the past fifty years is about as large of the value of growth in nonhealth goods and services. This makes clear that health care is about very substantial economic benefits, not just about economic costs. It helps make a persuasive case for future investment in health-related research and development. It also suggests that the future demand for health care will be substantial and that there will be a powerful appetite for interventions that preserve the quality of later life, including anti-ageing medicines.

The thirteenth international congress on anti-ageing medicine took place in December 2005 in Las Vegas, with more than five thousand attendees. The organisers claim that 'anti-ageing doctors earn more money than any other new medical speciality'. However, in the view of most reputable scientists involved in ageing research, claims for the success of such medical interventions are premature [23]. There is nevertheless considerable excitement in this rapidly developing area of research, with, for example, a variety of genetic modifications and other interventions in experimental animal models that extend longevity (see, for example, EMBO reports [24]).

Therefore, the possibility is that scientific advances could lead to significantly extended human life spans, conceivably well beyond the maximum natural age of about one hundred twenty years. Were this to prove feasible, at least two ethical questions would arise. First, would it be right to permit such a society to come about? The immediate response is that it would be difficult to prevent, given that each advance in treatment would serve to preserve human life, the traditional purpose of medicine. A second ethical question concerns who benefits and who pays. Expenditure on cosmetic surgery for beautification or rejuvenation cannot be justified within the National Health Service. Such treatments are therefore confined to those willing to pay out of their own pockets. But anti-ageing treatments that extend quality of life could be hard to deny to all and would add to the cost of the publicly funded health service, on top of the increase that would occur in any event. The question is how large a share of national expenditure could be pre-empted by a tax-funded health service in the long run and, if the limit to funding via taxation were to be reached so that the better-off purchased anti-ageing treatments out of their own resources, whether the resulting increase in inequality of life expectancy would be acceptable.

In contrast to such challenging ethical issues, preventative measures of the kind discussed in the present volume are uncontentious: nutrition, exercise, mental and social activity, and supportive physical and social environments. To which may be added measures to enhance mobility, the loss of which is a major cause of loss of quality of life in old age [25,26].

All these promote what is variously known as 'ageing well', 'successful ageing', or 'healthy ageing'. Certainly, if we regard ageing as taking place across the whole life course, then the idea of ageing well has real meaning.

But if we focus on ageing as a biological process that leads to frailty and death, then ageing well is perhaps more a matter of prolonging the years of middle age. Ageing well is unlike 'growing up well'. A healthy childhood should be followed by a healthy adult life. But healthy ageing is inevitably followed by decline and death. The question is: Can the choices we make influence the ultimate trajectory of decline, for good or ill?

Relevant to this question are a couple of 'comforting' concepts. One such concept that has had considerable currency is the 'compression of morbidity' hypothesis. The original proposition was that if longevity was more or less fixed, then efforts to postpone the onset of age-related disease would be rewarded by the compression of such conditions into a shorter period towards the end of life [27]. A second, related concept based on clinical observation is that of 'postponement as prevention'. It is argued that, because of age-associated loss of adaptability, the older we are when struck by a potentially disabling disease, such as stroke or coronary disease, the more likely we are to die rapidly rather than linger in a disabled state [28]. Thus, postponing disease, whether through lifestyle choices or preventative measures such as vaccination, should have the effect of compressing morbidity.

The current rapid increase in life expectancy at age sixty and above indicates that longevity is not fixed, however. Hence, compression of morbidity would only arise if healthy life expectancy—expected years of life in good or fairly good general health—is rising faster than life expectancy. Good-quality U.S. data indicate that the average health of the older population has been improving in recent years [29], likely due to a combination of improved medical treatment, behavioural change, increased use of assistive devices, and less exposure to disease in childhood [30]. Fries [31] argues that since the rate of decline of disability amongst older Americans at about 2% a year is faster than the rate of decline of mortality (1%), compression of morbidity is in fact occurring.

Analysis of U.K. data, on the other hand, suggests that healthy life expectancy has not been increasing as fast as has total life expectancy, with the result that people appear to be living more years in poor health or with a limiting long-standing illness—in effect a 'decompression of morbidity' [32]. This conclusion is based on surveys of self-perceived health status (unlike the U.S. data mentioned earlier, which relates to chronic disability assessed by the ability to perform activities of daily living). However, levels of self-reported heath can change over time for a number of reasons: changes in individuals' expectations of what is good health; economic incentives that persuade people to present themselves as ill; improvements in the diagnosis and detection of chronic conditions; as well as real changes in the population's health—for instance, the substitution of short-course, high-incidence acute disease (such as infectious disease) by longer course, lower incidence chronic conditions [33].

Thus, it is unclear at present whether the position in the United Kingdom is different from that in the United States as regards the compression of morbidity. But given the steady rise in life expectancy, as well as the considerable anecdotal evidence that many people over the age of sixty are adopting lively lifestyles rather than passive retirement [16], it is perhaps unlikely that late life morbidity in the United Kingdom is becoming more extensive. Rather, it is more probable that the extra years of life are, in effect, years of active middle age, rather than years of decrepitude at the end of the life course. From this viewpoint, the ageing well prescription offers the possibility of extending the period of healthy midlife. But do the choices we make whilst ageing well, or before, influence the ultimate trajectory of decline, for better or worse?

The incidence in the population of many diseases common in old age varies with socioeconomic factors. This implies determinants of disease that are substantially under individual or societal control, which means that if we are aware and well motivated we can hope to age well. Paying attention to diet, exercise, social engagement, and avoiding smoking all serve to reduce the risk of major age-associated conditions such as cardiovascular disease and depression [34]. However, it is not clear that all age-associated illnesses will be so reduced.

For instance, a substantial study [35] of the relationship between cognitive function and ageing has employed identical methodology for five diverse populations across the United Kingdom in two rural and three urban sites, each with different risk patterns and mortality rates. The incidence of dementia rises with age, and it is estimated that approximately one hundred eighty thousand new cases occur in England and Wales each year. Although many risk factors have been suggested for dementia and Alzheimer's disease, there is no evidence from this particular study that variation at population level in these risk factors influences incidence in the population. Thus, it is not clear that adopting the ageing well programme is likely to lessen one's chances of suffering from dementia in later life—a pessimistic inference that would justify further research effort.

A second instance of the likely lack of relationship between ageing well actions and age-associated illness is suggested by a study of visual impairment in a large sample of people age seventy-five and over in the United Kingdom, where no correlation was found with all-cause and cardiovascular mortality [36], although smoking was found to be a risk factor for age-related macular degeneration [37]. The implication is that, whilst stopping smoking would reduce the risk of loss of vision in old age, the other components of the ageing well agenda may not help.

Thus, if we live cleanly through midlife, aiming to age well, we can expect to reduce the incidence of many age-associated conditions but probably not of all. On the available evidence, we could hope to lessen the chances of sudden death due to ischaemic heart disease, thus staying alive potentially to suffer a slow decline of cognitive and visual functions. This is why the idea of ageing well is not entirely unproblematic.

Functional decline

Obviously, if we manage to avoid dying of one illness, we will die of some other. This is the concept of 'substitute mortality' [38]. The interesting question is whether in practice we have any choices. Could we influence prospectively the pattern of functional decline at the end of life? Are there actions we could take as part of an ageing well agenda or, even contrary to that, that would secure preferred outcomes? Bearing in mind that this last year of the life course is the period for which health-care expenditure is at its greatest, could these resources be more effectively deployed?

End of life decline has not been the subject of much research in recent years, although this topic has been the focus for the development of clinical practice. Nevertheless, some clinical observations suggest the existence of different trajectories of functional decline prior to death. A study of such decline deduced from Medicare claims in the United States showed that most of the data could be fitted into four predominant patterns [39,40]:

About one fifth of those who die, mostly cancer patients, experience fairly rapid decline.

Another fifth, mostly organ failure patients, experience long-term limitations with intermittent exacerbations and sudden death.

Two fifths face prolonged dwindling, as from frailty, disabling stroke, or dementia.

The remaining fifth die suddenly or cannot be simply classified.

Lunney et al. [41] then used an established cohort study, based on a sample of over four thousand decedents, to reconstruct patterns of functional decline in the months prior to death, measured by the ability to perform activities of daily living, and found that they could indeed be grouped largely into the four previously identified trajectories. Thus, it appears that there are different empirical patterns of functional decline, with functionality maintained at a high level in the case of those dying suddenly.

It is the geriatrician who is concerned with the medical care appropriate to the last part of life. Geriatric medicine is numerically a strong speciality in Britain, more so than in other countries. Arguably, this has arisen not only because of the undoubted skills and values of the speciality, but also because a monolithic National Health Service has in the past given older patients limited choice of where to be treated. But we are now moving into a new era in which 'patient choice' is the watchword. People might not naturally elect to seek the services of a geriatrician if it seems that a specialist is better able to treat their current condition. If geriatric medicine is to have a future in an era of patient choice, it will be in helping us manage the trajectory of decline of body and of mind [42].

Conclusion

This symposium was the forty-seventh in the annual series arranged by the Society for the Study of Human Biology. It was only the second to deal primarily with ageing. Arguably, given the centrality of ageing to human existence, as well as the good progress being made in understanding the biology of ageing in model systems, some greater focus by human biologists on late life events would be well justified.

In carrying forward the development of policy and practice, we could usefully consider a two-part objective for focusing research priorities. First, we need to generate the evidence that will help maximise high-quality years of life over the whole life course. Many of the chapters in this volume are very relevant to this first element of the objective. But at the same time, we also need to maximise the quality of life in the final years of life, the second part of the objective. How to achieve this double objective is the challenge. Optimists will hope that evidence for a declining trend in disability in old age means that the period of late life morbidity is being compressed in duration, the result of people adopting the 'ageing well' agenda. Pessimists can worry, amongst other things, about a possible rise in incidence of dementia. At present, we are short of the evidence needed to understand what is happening and to make good decisions.

The final period of life is as much a part of the human life course as any other. It has been neglected as a subject for study, for perhaps understandable reasons: complexity, distaste, and difficulty in investigating. Yet we surely need to understand more if we are to aspire to exercise, in this final phase, the control we expect to have at earlier stages.

References

1. Government Actuary's Department, National Population Projections 2004-based, London, 2005.
2. Vaupel, J., Setting the stage: A generation of centenarians? *Washington Q*, Summer, 197–200, 2000.
3. Oeppen, J. and Vaupel, J.W., Broken limits to life expectancy, *Science*, 296, 1029–1031, 2002.
4. Olshansky, S.J. et al., A potential decline in life expectancy in the United States in the 21st century, *N Engl J Med*, 352, 1138–1145, 2005.
5. Pensions Commission, A new pension settlement for the twenty-first century; the second report of the Pensions Commission, http://www.pensionscommission.org.uk/, 2005.
6. Department for Work and Pensions, Security in retirement: Towards a new pensions system, Cm 6841, May 2006.
7. Population Ageing Associates, Ageing Assets—Implications of population ageing for the South East Region, http://www.ageconcern.org.uk/AgeConcern/about_5066.htm, October 2005.
8. Department of Health, Working lives; flexible retirement: Guidance for managers, London, November 2001.

9. Department for Work and Pensions, Older workers: Statistical information booklet, London, Spring 2005.
10. Ilmarinen, J.E., Aging workers, *Occupational Environ Med*, 58, 546–552, 2001.
11. Costa, G., Goedhard, W., and Ilmarinen, J. (eds.), *Assessment and Promotion of Workability, Health and Well-being of Ageing Workers*, Elsevier, London, 2005.
12. Rowe, J.W. and Kahn, R.L., *Successful Aging*, Dell, New York, 1999.
13. Peters, M., Cressy, R., and Storey, D., The economic impact of ageing on entrepreneurship and SMEs, Forward Studies Unit, European Commission, Brussels, 1999.
14. Galenson, D.W., The life cycles of modern artists: Theory, measurement and implications, NBER Working Paper 9539, National Bureau for Economic Research, Cambridge, MA, 2003.
15. Galenson, D.W., *Artistic Capital*, Routledge, London, 2006.
16. Metz, D. and Underwood, M., *Older Richer Fitter: Identifying the Customer Needs of Britain's Ageing Population*, Age Concern Books, London, 2005.
17. Stroud, D., *The 50-Plus Market*, Kogan Page, London, 2005.
18. Metz, D., Can the impact of ageing on health care costs be avoided? *J Health Serv Res Policy*, 4, 249–252, 1999.
19. Spillman, B.C. and Lubitz, J., The effect of longevity on spending for acute and long-term care, *N Engl J Med*, 342, 1409–1415, 2000.
20. Mcgrail, K., Green, B., Barer, M.L., Evans, R.G., Hertzman, C., and Normand, C., Age, costs of acute and long-term care and proximity to death: Evidence for 1987–88 and 1994–95 in British Columbia, *Age Ageing*, 29, 249–253, 2000.
21. OECD in Figures, 2005 edition, OECD, Paris, 2005.
22. Nordhaus, W.D., The health of nations: The contribution of improved health to living standards. In: *Measuring the Gains from Medical Research: An Economic Approach*, ed. Murphy, K. and Topel, T., University of Chicago Press, Chicago, 2003.
23. Olshansky, S.J., Hayflick, L., and Carnes, B.A., No truth to the fountain of youth, *Scientific Am*, June 2002.
24. EMBO reports, vol 6, Special Issue on the science of ageing and anti-ageing, July 2005.
25. Metz, D., Mobility of older people and their quality of life, *Transport Policy*, 7, 149–152, 2000.
26. Metz, D., Transport policy for an ageing population, *Transport Rev*, 23, 375–386, 2003.
27. Fries, J.F., Aging, natural death, and the compression of morbidity. *N Engl J Med*, 303, 130–135, 1980.
28. Evans, J.G., Implications for health services in ageing: Science, medicine and society, *Phil Trans R Soc Lond B*, 352, 1887–1893, 1997.
29. Manton, K.G. and Gu, X., Changes in the prevalence of chronic disability in the United States black and nonblack population above age 65 from 1982 to 1999, *Proc Nat Acad Sci USA*, 98, 6354–6359, 2001.
30. Cutler, D.M., The reduction in disability among the elderly, *Proc Nat Acad Sci USA*, 98, 6546–6547, 2001.
31. Fries, J.F., Measuring and monitoring success in compressing morbidity, *Ann Intern Med*, 139, 455–459, 2003.
32. Kelly, S., Baker, A., and Gupta, S., Healthy life expectancy in Great Britain, 1980–96, and its use as an indicator in United Kingdom government strategies, *Health Stat Q*, 7, 32–37, Autumn, 2000.

33. Office for National Statistics, Evidence to House of Lords Science and Technology Committee enquiry, Ageing: Scientific aspects, vol. 1 report para 2.21, The Stationery Office, London, July 2005.
34. Ebrahim, S. and Kalache, A. (eds.), *Epidemiology in Old Age*, BMJ Publishing, London, 1996.
35. Matthews, F., Brayne, C., et al., The incidence of dementia in England and Wales: Findings from the five identical sites of the MRC CFA study, *Public Library Sci Med*, 2, 0753–0763, 2005.
36. Thiagarajan, M., Evans, J.R., Smeeth, L., Wormald, R.P.L., and Fletcher, A.E., Cause-specific visual impairment and mortality: Results from a population-based study of older people in the United Kingdom, *Arch Opthalmol*, 123, 1397–1403, 2005.
37. Evans, J.R., Fletcher, A.E., and Wormald, R.P.L., 28,000 Cases of age-related macular degeneration causing visual loss in people age 75 and above in the United Kingdom may be attributable to smoking, *Br J Opthalmol*, 85, 550–553, 2005.
38. Van de Water, H.P.A., Health expectancy and the problem of substitute morbidity, *Phil Trans R Soc Lond B*, 352, 1819–1827, 1997.
39. Lunney, J.R., Lynn, J., and Hogan, C., Profiles of older Medicare decedents, *J Am Geriatr Soc*, 50, 1108–1112, 2002.
40. Lynn, J. and Adamson, D.M., Living well at the end of life: Adapting health care to serious chronic illness in old age, RAND Health, Santa Monica, CA, 2003.
41. Lunney, J.R., Lynn, J., Foley, D.F., Lipson, S., and Guralnick, J.M., Patterns of functional decline at the end of life, *JAMA*, 289, 2387–2392, 2003.
42. Metz, D.H. and LaBrooy, S.J., The future of geriatric medicine in an era of patient choice, *Age Ageing*, 34, 553–555, 2005.

Index

A

Aberdeen studies, *see* Scottish Mental surveys
Acheson's committee, 79
Active minds, 147
Activities of daily living (ADLs), 86
Actuary Department, 155–156
Acute care costs, 121–122
Adaptive responses, cognitive function, 54
ADLs, *see* Activities of daily living (ADLs)
Aedo studies, 3, 127–136
Age-related macular degeneration (AMD)
    antioxidants, 28–30
    cataracts, 26
    dietary factors, 28–31
    fats, 30–31
    fundamentals, 25–27, 31
    genetic susceptibility, 28
    light exposure, 27
    risk factors, 27–31
    smoking, 27
Age-related maculopathy (ARM), 27, 29
Agreeableness, 55–56
Air pollution, winter deaths, 105–106
Alameda cohort study, 73
Alcohol
    HALE study, 8
    minimum income for healthy living, 149
    survival chances, 2
Alpha carotene, 60, *see also* Beta carotene; Carotenoids
Alzheimer's disease
    genetic studies, 58
    incidence, 161
    physical activity protection, 19
    vitamin B_{12}, 10
Ancestry impact, living arrangements, 93
Ankle support, 21

Anti-ageing treatments and doctors, 159
Antioxidants, 28–30, 54
Apoptosis, 54
Arachidonic acid, 61
AREDS trial, 30
Argentina, 127
ARM, *see* Age-related maculopathy (ARM)
Artistic creativity, 157–158
Assessment, *see* Intervention cost-effectiveness assessment (CEA)
Attentiveness, reminiscence, 41
Austria, 93
Automobile ownership, 75–76, 148–149

B

Balance, 144, *see also* Physical activity
Barriers
    exercise, 19–21
    reminiscence, 42–43
Bath and Deeg studies, 96
Bathing, caregiver's role, 44, 48
Beaver Dam Eye Study, 29
Behaviour
    risky, 69
    winter deaths, 105–106
Belgium, 7
Bending, 144, *see also* Physical activity
Benefits, reminiscence, 40–42
Benzodiazepine use, 18
Berlin Ageing Study, 96
Beta carotene, 29–30, *see also* Alpha carotene; Carotenoids
Beveridge studies, 149
Bicycling, 148
Biography
    assumption, 47

using, 36
Birth rates, 86–91
Black Report, 68
Blue light
    cataract and AMD risk factors, 27
    eye health, 28
Bornat studies, 48
Bowling and Grundy studies, 96
Breeze studies, 3, 67–80
Butler studies, 36

C

Cancer
    cognitive function, 62–63
    physical activity protection, 19
CAPH, *see* London School of Hygiene and
        Tropical Medicine Centre for
        Ageing and Public Health
        (CAPH)
Cardiovascular disease, 79, *see also* Heart
        disease
Caregivers and caregiving, *see also* Family
        support
    acute care costs, 121–122
    bathing, 44, 48
    caring role, 44–45
    chatting, 44, 48
    couples, 121
    economic perspectives, 121
    intervention cost-effectiveness
        assessment, 133–134
    measurement and valuation, 133–134
    reminiscence impact, 36
Care homes, reminiscence, 47–48
Carotenoids
    antioxidants, 30
    eye health, 28–29
Car ownership, 75–76, 148–149
Catalase, 28
Cataracts
    antioxidants, 28–30
    cataracts, 26
    dietary factors, 28–31
    eye diseases, 26
    fats, 30–31
    fundamentals, 25–26, 31
    genetic susceptibility, 28
    light exposure, 27
    risk factors, 27–31
    smoking, 27
Cathy (comments), 45
CEA, *see* Intervention cost-effectiveness
        assessment (CEA)

CENEX Chile study, 3, 131–133
Central European countries, 120
Centre for Ageing and Public Health, *see*
        London School of Hygiene and
        Tropical Medicine Centre for
        Ageing and Public Health
        (CAPH)
Cezanne (artist), 157–158
Challenges, reminiscence, 47
Chatting, caregiver's role, 44, 48
Cheston studies, 36
Childhood (initial) intelligence value
    cognitive function, 53
    dementia, 57
    fundamentals, 3, 52
    genetic studies, 58–59
    health-related behaviors, 61
    risk factor, 57
    stability, 56–57
Children, contact levels, 94
Chile nutrition programme, 3, 131–133
Cholesterol
    cognitive function, 60
    dementia, 2
Choriocapillaris, 27
Chung studies, 35–49
Cobalamin, *see* Vitamin B_{12}
Cochrane Review, 11
Cognitive function
    adaptive responses, 54
    childhood (initial) intelligence value, 53
    cognitive reserve, 53–54
    compensatory responses, 54
    dementia threshold, 53–54
    diet, 3
    food supplements, 3
    fundamentals, 3, 51–52, 63
    genetic studies, molecular, 58–59
    health checks, 3
    health-related behaviors, 61–63
    key principles, 53
    maximum or optimal, 53–54
    molecular genetic studies, 58–59
    nutritional studies, 59–61
    personality role, 55–56
    reserve, 53–54
    risk factors, 57
    Scottish Mental surveys, 56–63
    smoking, 3
    vascular disease risks, 3
    vitamins, 3
Cognitive reserve, 53–54
Coleman studies, 46–47
Collins studies, 106
Comfort zone, 43, 47

Community kitchens, 127
Compensatory responses, 54
Compression of morbidity, 160–161
Comrades, discontinuity, 42–43
Conscientiousness, 56
Constructing familiarity, 37
Consumption, commercial, 158
Contacts, 93–94
Contingencies, 149
Copenhagen City Heart Study, 96
Cosmetic surgery, 159
Cost-benefit analysis, 130
Cost-effectiveness assessment (CEA), *see*
      Intervention cost-effectiveness
      assessment (CEA)
Cost-minimisation analysis, 130
Cost-utility analysis, 130
Couch potatoes, 20, *see also* Exercise; Physical
      activity
Couples, 121, *see also* Marital status
Creativity, 157–158

D

Dangour studies, 1–4, 139–151
Debit cards, food purchases, 127
Deeg, Bath and, studies, 96
Deeming studies, 139–151
De Groot studies, 2, 5–11
Dementia
    cholesterol, 2
    cognitive function, 53–54, 57
    genetics, 58
    incidence, 161
    physical activity, 2, 19
    vitamin B_{12}, 10
    weight, 2
Demographics
    contacts, 93–94
    family support, 91–98
    fundamentals, 85–86
    future trends, 98–99
    intergenerational co-residence, 91, 93
    kin networks, 86–91
    living arrangements, 91, 93
    projections, 85
    provision of support, 93–94
Denmark
    bicycling, 148
    contact levels, 93
    family support, 96, 98
    SENECA, 7
Denominator, cost-effectiveness analysis, 130
Dental care, 146

Depression, 18–19
Determinants, exercise, 19–21
DHA (docosahexaenoic acid), 30
Diabetes
    physical activity protection, 19
    retinopathy, 26
Diet, *see also* Nutrition
    antioxidants, 30
    cognitive function, 3
    eye diseases, 28–31
    fat, 30–31
    income impact, 141–142
    minimum income for healthy living, 141
    patterns, nutritional concerns, 8
    SENECA study, 8
Disability-adjusted life-years (DALYs), 130
Discontinuity, 42–43
Discussion, reminiscence, 46–48
Diseases, 161, *see also* Infections; *specific*
    disease
Dislocation feelings, 43
Docosahexaenoic acid (DHA), 30, 61
Donaldson studies, 135
Downward transfers, 91
Dry age-related macular degeneration (dry
    AMD), 26

E

Eastern European countries
    fertility rates, 87
    unemployment, 120
Ebrahim and Smith studies, 79
Economic perspectives
    caregiving, 121
    evaluation role, 129–130
    financial perspective comparison,
        124–125
    fundamentals, 117–118, 125–126
    health needs, 121–122
    pension issue, 122–124
    social care, 121–122
    work, 118–120
Edinburgh studies, *see* Scottish Mental
      surveys
Edna (comments), 41
Education impact
    cognitive function, 54–55
    dementia, 57
    health inequalities, 69
    longevity implications, 156
    risk factor, 57
    socioeconomic position, 73
Elford studies, 35–49

Elsie (comments), 44
Endurance exercise, 20
Energy efficiency
    fundamentals, 103–104
    housing role, 106–107
    mortality, 104
    nutritional concerns, 10–11
    pathophysiological mechanisms, 105–106
    policy implications, 112–113
    socioeconomic variations, 110
    temperature, 104
English House Conditions Survey (EHCS),
        107, 145
English Longitudinal Survey of Ageing
        (2002)
    contact levels, 93
    family support, 97
Environmental influences
    cognitive function, 54
    housing, 3
    meal ambience, 11, 60
    preferred guidelines, 6
Equitable Life case, 123
Erikson studies, 36
Ethnicity, living arrangements, 93
Europe, 106, *see also* specific area
Everyday talk, 38, 40–42
Exclusions, income impact, 149
Exercise, *see also* Physical activity
    barriers, 19–21
    determinants, 19–21
    fundamentals, 2, 17–18, 21–22
    minimum income for healthy living, 142,
        144
    physical activity comparison, 18–19
    safety, 19–21
Expenditure and Food Surveys, 141, 145, 149
Experiences, openness to, 56
Extraversion, 56
Eye Disease Case Control Study, 29
Eye health
    age-related macular degeneration, 26–31
    antioxidants, 28–30
    cataracts, 26
    dietary factors, 28–31
    fats, 30–31
    fundamentals, 2, 25–26, 31
    genetic susceptibility, 28
    light exposure, 27
    ophthalmic services, 146
    smoking, 27
    visual impairment, 161

F

Falling mortality rates, 89–90
Familiarity, constructing, 37
Family folklore, 41–42
Family support, *see also* Caregivers and
        caregiving; Kin networks
    demographics, 91–98
    fundamentals, 3
Fats, dietary, 30–31
Feelings
    dislocation, 43
    valued, 40–41
Fertility rates, 86–91
Financial perspectives, 124–125
Findings
    reminiscence, 46–48
    socioeconomic impact, 70–78
Finland
    dementia, 2
    work ability, 157
Finland, Italy, the Netherlands Elderly
        (FINE) study, 7
Fish and fish oil
    cognitive function, 61
    preferred guidelines, 6
Fletcher studies, 1–4, 25–31, 139–151
Flexibility, 144, *see also* Physical activity
Fluid intake, 6
Folate, 10, *see also* Vitamin B_{12}
Food
    access, 11, 59
    community kitchens, 127
    debit cards, 127
    feeding assistance, 11
    flavours, 11
    food baskets, 127
    policy implications, 79
    preferred nutritional approach, 3
Food supplements, 3, 52, *see also* Nutrition;
        specific type
Formal care, 133–134
Fractures, 9–10
Frailty, nutritional concerns, 10–11
France
    demographic projections, 85
    mortality and temperature, 104
    SENECA, 7
Fred (comments), 43
Friends, discontinuity, 42–43
Fries studies, 160
Froggatt studies, 37
Fruit and fruit juice
    antioxidants, 30
    preferred guidelines, 6

Fuel costs, 112–113
Future research and trends
   demographics, 98–99
   intervention cost-effectiveness
      assessment, 135–136

G

GA age-related macular degeneration
   (GAAMD), 26
GAAMD, *see* Geographic atrophy age-related
   macular degeneration (GAAMD)
Gait, slow, 18
Galenson studies, 157–158
Gambling, 149
Gaps, income impact, 149
Gender
   cognitive function, 57
   contact levels, 94
   demographic projections, 86
   disabling health problems, 86
   family support, 96
   life expectancy, 87
   marriage rates, 87, 89
   minimum income for healthy living,
      140–141
   social housing transition, 78
   socioeconomic position, 70–71, 73, 76
Genealogy, 41–42
Genetics
   cognitive function, 54, 58–59
   eye diseases, 28
   influence, 18
Geographic atrophy age-related macular
   degeneration (GAAMD), 26
Geriatric medicine, 162
Germany, 85
Giddens studies, 46
Glaucoma, 26
Glutathione, 28
Glutathione peroxidase, 28
Goldblatt studies, 75
Goudie studies, 35–49
Government Actuary Department, 155–156
Grains, 30
Grundy, Bowling and, studies, 96
Grundy studies, 1–4, 85–99

H

HALE, *see* Healthy Ageing: a Longitudinal
   Study in Europe (HALE)
Hazard exposure, 69
Health and Lifestyle Study, 73

Health care
   costs, 3
   dementia, 57
   income impact, 146
Health checks, 3
Health gain, 129
Health inequalities
   findings, 70–78
   fundamentals, 3, 67–68
   longitudinal studies, 75
   middle age socioeconomic position, 70–73
   policy implications, 78–80
   socioeconomic position theories, 68–78
   source data, 70
   study considerations, 67–68
   transitions in status, 76, 78
Health needs, 121–122
Health Professionals Study, 29–30
Health-related behaviors, 61–63
Health-related quality of life (HRQOL)
   measures, 135
Health Surveys for England, 141
Healthy Ageing: a Longitudinal Study in
   Europe (HALE), 6–8
Healthy eating index (HEI), 30
Hearing impairment, 42
Heart disease
   physical activity protection, 19
   policy implications, 79
   socioeconomic position, 72
HEI, *see* Healthy eating index (HEI)
Hinchliff studies, 35–49
Holland, 148
Home Health and Safety Rating System, 113
Homeostatic control, 10
Homocysteine
   cognitive function, 60
   vitamin B_{12}, 10
Homozygosity, 28
Honolulu cohort study, 73
Hospital Anxiety Depression Scale, 57
Hospital occupancy, 67
Household chores, 21, 78
House of Commons Select Committee on
   Social Security, 140
Housing, *see also* Temperature
   energy efficiency, 106–107
   environment, 3
   health inequalities, 69
   hygiene, 147–148
   income impact, 144–145, 147–148
   indoor temperature, 3
   management, 78
   property condition, 107
   quality, 3

social housing transition, 76
HRQOL (health-related quality of life)
        measures, 135
Hygiene, 147–148
Hypertension, 62

I

Improving energy intake, 10–11
Income impact
    active minds, 147
    cognitive function, 62
    contingencies, 149
    diet, 141–142
    exclusions, 149
    fundamentals, 140, 150–151
    gaps, 149
    health care, 146
    home hygiene, 147–148
    housing, 144–145
    hygiene, 147–148
    inefficiencies, 149
    methods, 141
    mind activity, 147
    personal hygiene, 147–148
    physical activity, 142, 144
    population study, 140–149
    psychosocial relations, 147
    results, 141–149
    self-reported quality, 79
    social inclusion, 147
    socioeconomic position, 73
    transportation, 148–149
    variations, 149
Individual nonhealth benefits, 129
Inefficiencies, 149
Inequalities studies, 67–68
Infections
    life expectancy, 156
    winter deaths, 105–106
Inflammatory response, 54
Influences
    health and disease, 18
    socioeconomic impact, 75–78
Influenza, winter deaths, 105–106
Informal care, 133–134
Initial (childhood) intelligence value
    cognitive function, 53
    dementia, 57
    fundamentals, 3, 52
    genetic studies, 58–59
    health-related behaviors, 61
    risk factor, 57
    stability, 56–57

Injuries, *see* Safety
Institutionalised situations, 10–11
Intellectual traits, stability, 56
Intensity of activities, 18
Intergenerational co-residence, 91, 93
Intergenerational talk, 38–42, 47
Intertemporal transfers of rights, 123
Intervention cost-effectiveness assessment
        (CEA)
    caregivers, 133–134
    Chile nutrition programme, 131–133
    economic evaluation role, 129–130
    elements of, 130–133
    fundamentals, 3, 136
    future research, 135–136
    methological issues, 127–129, 133–135
    objectives, specific, 129
    outcomes, 134–135
    policy priorities, 135–136
    specific objectives, 129
Ireland, 93
Italy
    demographic projections, 85
    SENECA, 7

J

Jane (comments), 40, 44
Japan
    demographic projections, 85
    fertility rates, 87
    living arrangements, 93
Jean (comments), 44
Joan (comments), 43
John (comments), 40–41
Johri studies, 136

K

Kawachi, Woodward and, studies, 68
Keady, Nolan and, studies, 36
Keatinge studies, 106
'Keepers,' *see* Family folklore
Kenyon, Randall and, studies, 37
Key principles, cognitive function, 53
Kin networks, *see also* Family support
    demographics, 86–91
    fundamentals, 3

L

Latin America, 127
Leisure pursuits, *see* Recreational pursuits

Lens Opacities Case Control Study, 29
Lewinter studies, 36
Lifestyle
    influence, 18
    nutritional concerns, 8
Light, *see also* Vitamin D
    antioxidants, 29
    cataract and AMD risk factor, 27
Linguistic ability, 57
Link and Phelan studies, 79
Linoleic acid, 30
Listening, 41
Living arrangements
    demographics, 91, 93
    South Africa, 135
London, England, 104
London School of Hygiene and Tropical
        Medicine Centre for Ageing and
        Public Health (CAPH), 2
Longevity
    functional decline, 162
    fundamentals, 1, 3–4, 163
    health, 158–161
    implications, 156–158
    increasing, 155–156
Longitudinal Study, 70–78
Lubitz studies, 128
Lunney studies, 162
Lutein
    dietary fats, 31
    eye health, 28–29

M

Maria (comments), 40
Marital status
    caregiving, 121
    contact levels, 94
Marriage rates, 87, 89
Mary (comments), 41, 45
McIntyre studies, 96
McKee studies, 3, 35–49
McKiernan, Woods and, studies, 36
McMurdo studies, 2, 17–22
Meals
    ambience and social context, 11, 60
    preferred guidelines, 6
Meat, 30
Medicare claims, United States, 162
Mediterranean style diet
    HALE study, 8
    survival chances, 2
Mellowing, personality, 56
Memory loss, 42

Metabolic equivalents (METs), 18
Methods
    income impact, 141
    intervention cost-effectiveness
        assessment, 127–129, 133–135
    reminiscence, 37–38
METs, *see* Metabolic equivalents (METs)
Metz studies, 3, 155–163
Mexico City, 127
Micronutrient intake, 105–106
Middle age socioeconomic position, 70–73
MIDSPAN studies, 62
Milk and milk products, 30
Milne studies, 11
Mind activity, 147
Minimum income for healthy living (MIHL)
    active minds, 147
    cognitive function, 62
    contingencies, 149
    diet, 141–142
    exclusions, 149
    fundamentals, 140, 150–151
    gaps, 149
    health care, 146
    home hygiene, 147–148
    housing, 144–145
    hygiene, 147–148
    inefficiencies, 149
    methods, 141
    mind activity, 147
    personal hygiene, 147–148
    physical activity, 142, 144
    population study, 140–149
    psychosocial relations, 147
    results, 141–149
    self-reported quality, 79
    social inclusion, 147
    socioeconomic position, 73
    transportation, 148–149
    variations, 149
Misconceptions, exercise, 20
Mobility
    minimum income for healthy living, 144
    socioeconomic position, 75
Molecular genetic studies, 58–59
MONICA surveys, 60
Monitoring insufficiency, 79
Moray House Test, 56
Morbidity, compression of, 160–161
Morris studies, 3, 139–151
Mortality
    nutritional concerns, 8
    temperature impact, 104
Mortality, substitute, 162

MRC Trile of the Assessment and
    Management of People (MRC
    Study), 70
MRI measures and investigations, 57, 60
Muscle mass, *see also* Physical activity
    minimum income for healthy living, 144
    physical decline, 19

N

National Health Service, 157, 159, 162
National Institute of Ageing Working Group
    on Ageing and Genetic
    Epidemiology, 53
National Service Framework, 67
NEO-FF Personality Scale, 57
Neovascular age-related macular
    degeneration (NVAMD), 26,
    29–30
Neuroticism, 56
Newton studies, 37
Nolan and Keady studies, 36
Nolan studies, 36
'No pain, no gain' phrase, 21
Nordhaus studies, 158
Nordic countries, 93
Normand, Charles, 3, 117–126
North America
    family support, 98
    living arrangements, 93
    mobility, 75
Northern European countries
    contact levels, 93–94
    family support, 98
Northwest European countries, 93
Numerator, cost-effectiveness analysis, 130
Nurses Health Study, 28–30
Nutrition, *see also* Diet
    cognitive function, 59–61
    dietary patterns, 8
    energy balance and intake, 10–11
    frailty, 10–11
    fundamentals, 2, 5–6, 11
    HALE study, 6–8
    improving energy intake, 10–11
    influence, 18
    institutionalised situations, 10–11
    lifestyle, 8
    mortality, 8
    SENECA study, 6–8
    vitamin B_{12}, 9–10
    vitamin D, 8–9
NVAMD, *see* Neovascular age-related
    macular degeneration (NVAMD)

O

Obesity
    decline predictor, 18
    life expectancy, 156
Objectives, specific, 129
Occupation
    cognitive function, 54–55
    dementia, 57
    socioeconomic position, 73
    working, 118–120
Ogg and Renault studies, 94
Olausson studies, 73
Omega-3 fatty acids, 31, 61
Omega-6 fatty acids, 61
Ophthalmic services, 146, *see also* Eye health
Orderliness, 56
Osteoporosis, 19
Outcomes
    economic evaluation, 129–131
    measurement and valuation, 134–135
Overload, 44–45
Over-the-counter medicines, 146

P

PACAM (Programme for Complementary
    Food in Older People), 131–132
Paisley, Scotland, *see* MIDSPAN studies
Parental marital status, 94
Pathophysiological mechanisms, 105–106
Patronisation, 45
Payton, Reed and, studies, 37, 48
Pensions
    economic perspectives, 122–124
    insufficiency, 3
    longevity implications, 156
    working, 119
Pensions Committee, 156
Performance, cognitive function, 53–54
Personal hygiene, 147–148
Personality, 55–57
Perspective, cost-effectiveness analysis, 130
Phelan, Link and, studies, 79
Philadelphia Geriatric Morale Scale, 70
Photoreceptors, 28
Physical activity, *see also* Exercise
    amount needed, 8, 19
    dementia, 2
    energy intake, increasing, 11
    exercise comparison, 18–19
    HALE study, 8
    income impact, 142, 144
    misconceptions, 20

present talk, 46
SENECA study, 8
survival chances, 2
walking, 8
Picasso (artist), 157
Platitudes, 45, 47
Policy
energy efficiency, 112–113
family support, 98
focus, 1
health inequalities, 78–80
intervention cost-effectiveness
assessment, 135–136
socioeconomic impact, 78–80
Pollution, air, 105–106
Population studies
disease incidence, 161
income impact, 140–149
survival ages, 6
Portugal, 7
Posterior subcapsular opacities (PSCs), 26
Poverty
cognitive function, 62
home heating, 110
Present talk, 46
Productivity, 120
Programmed cell death, 54
Programme for Complementary Food in
Older People (PACAM), 131–132
Property condition, 107, *see also* Housing
Provision of support, 93–94
PSCs, *see* Posterior subcapsular opacities
(PSCs)
Psychosocial relations
health and poverty impact, 69
income impact, 147
Public transportation, 148–149
Puentes studies, 36
Pulsford studies, 36

Q

Quality-adjusted life-years (QALYs), 130,
135–136

R

Randall and Kenyon studies, 37
Randomized controlled trials (RCTs), 30–31
RCTs, *see* Randomized controlled trials
(RCTs)
Reactive oxygen species (ROS), 27
REACT study, 30
Recreational pursuits

cognitive function, 54–55
dementia, 57
Redistributive system
financial *vs.* economic perspectives,
124–125
policy implications, 79
Reed and Payton studies, 37, 48
Refractive errors, 26
Relationships, *see* Social relationships
Religion, living arrangements, 93
Reminiscence
barriers, 42–43
benefits, 40–42
care homes, 47–48
caring role, 44–45
challenges, 47
comfort zone, 43
discontinuity, 42–43
discussion, 46–48
everyday talk, 38, 40–42
feeling valued, 40–41
findings, 46–48
fundamentals, 3, 36–37, 48
intergenerational links, 41–42
method, 37–38
overload, 44–45
present talk, 46
relationships, 38, 40
results, 38–46
self-identity, 46–47
significance, 40–41
tensions, 45–46
Renault, Ogg and, studies, 94
Renfew, Scotland, *see* MIDSPAN studies
Reserve, cognitive function, 53–54
Results
cost-effectiveness analysis, 131
income impact, 141–149
reminiscence, 38–46
Retinal pigment epithelium (RPE), 26–28
Retirement age, society's viewpoint, 118
Rigid personality, 56
Risk factors, cognitive function, 57
Roberts, Thorsheim and, studies, 36
Roman Catholic Church, 119
ROS, *see* Reactive oxygen species (ROS)
Rotterdam Study, 30
RPE, *see* Retinal pigment epithelium (RPE)
Rubenstein studies, 37

S

Safety
exercise, 20–21

housing maintenance, 144–145
Salt intake, 141
Sam (comments), 43
Sameness, 56
SAP, *see* Standard assessment procedure
    (SAP)
Scandinavia
    family support, 98
    housing role, 106
Scotland
    cognitive function, 62
    family support, 98
Scottish Council for Research in Education,
    56
Scottish Health Survey, 19–20
Scottish Mental surveys, 52, 56–63
Second World Assembly on Ageing, 127
SEIQoL (Structured Evaluation Inventory for
    Quality of Life), 57
Self-identity
    cognitive function, 56
    reminiscence, 36, 38, 46–47
SENECA, *see* Survey in Europe on Nutrition
    and the Elderly: a Concerted
    Approach (SENECA)
Sensitivity analysis, cost-effectiveness
    analysis, 131
Sequestration, 37
Set-in-ways type personality, 56
SF36 (quality of life measurement), 57
Shadow price, 133–134
SHARE (Survey of Health and Retirement in
    Europe), 93–94
Shoes, exercise safety, 21
Short-acting benzodiazepine use, 18
Siblings, contact levels, 94
Sickness Impact Profile, 70
Significance, reminiscence, 40–41
Slow gait, 18
Smith, Davey, 69
Smith, Ebrahim and, studies, 79
Smoking
    antioxidants, 29
    cognitive function, 3, 61–62
    eye diseases, 27, 161
    genetics, 28
    HALE study, 8
    minimum income for healthy living, 149
    SENECA study, 8
Social care, economic perspectives, 121–122
Social nonhealth benefits, 129
Social relationships
    cognitive function, 54
    eating context, 11, 60
    family support, 96

housing hygiene, 147–148
personality role, 55
reminiscence, 37
social death, 37
social housing transition, 76, 78
Society for the Study of Human Biology
    (SSHB), 2, 163
Socioeconomic impact
    disease incidence, 161
    findings, 70–78
    fundamentals, 3
    inequalities studies, 67–68
    influence, 75–78
    longitudinal studies, 75
    middle age socioeconomic position, 70–73
    policy implications, 78–80
    source data, 70
    theories, 68–69
    transitions in, 76–78
Socioeconomic variations, 110
Sophie (comments), 45
Source data, 70
South Africa, 135
Southern European countries
    contact levels, 93–94
    family support, 97
    fertility rates, 87
    living arrangements, 93
    SENECA, 9
Spain
    demographic projections, 85
    mobility, 75
    SENECA, 7
Specific objectives, 129
SSHB, *see* Society for the Study of Human
    Biology (SSHB)
Stability, 144, *see also* Physical activity
Staden studies, 48
Stamford Binet Test, 56
Standard assessment procedure (SAP), 107
Strength training, *see also* Physical activity
    minimum income for healthy living, 144
    muscle impact, 19
Stretching, 144, *see also* Physical activity
Structured Evaluation Inventory for Quality
    of Life (SEIQoL), 57
Study considerations, health inequalities,
    67–68
Substitute mortality, 162
Sunlight, *see also* Vitamin D
    antioxidants, 29
    cataract and AMD risk factor, 27
Superoxide dismutase, 28
Supplements, *see* Food supplements;
    Vitamins (general)

Survey in Europe on Nutrition and the Elderly: a Concerted Approach (SENECA), 6–9
Survey of Health and Retirement in Europe (SHARE), 93–94
Survival chances, 2
Sutherland Commission, 67
Sweden
    contact levels, 93
    socioeconomic position, 73
Switzerland, 7
Sylvia (comments), 42

T

Taiwan, 97
Taste sensitivity, 10–11, *see also* Food
Taxation, 124–125
Temperature
    indoor, 3
    mortality effects, 104
Tensions, reminiscence, 45–46
The Netherlands
    contact levels, 93
    SENECA, 7
Theories, socioeconomic impact, 68–69
Thorsheim and Roberts studies, 36
Transgenerational talk, *see* Intergenerational talk
Transitions in status, 76, 78
Transportation, 148–149
Twigg studies, 48
Twisting movements, 21

U

U.K. Department of Health, 68
Ultraviolet radiation (UVR), 27, *see also* Vitamin D
Unemployment, 120
United Nations Population Division, 127
United States
    eye health, 25
    family support, 96, 98
    Medicare claims, 162
    mobility, 75
    socioeconomic position, 73
Uses for Objects Test, 57

V

van Asselt studies, 9
Van der Wielen studies, 8

van Staveren studies, 2, 5–11
Variations, income impact, 149
Variety, resistance, 56
Vascular disease, 3, 62–63
VA (visual acuity), 25
VECAT study, 30
Vegetables
    antioxidants, 30
    preferred guidelines, 6
Vehicle ownership, 75–76, 148–149
Verticalisation, 90
Viewpoint, cost-effectiveness analysis, 130
Visual acuity (VA), 25
Visual impairment, 161
Vitamin A, 28
Vitamin B_{12}
    insufficient intake, 5
    minimum income for healthy living, 141
    nutritional concerns, 9–10
Vitamin C
    cognitive function, 60
    eye health, 28–30
Vitamin D
    insufficient intake, 5
    nutritional concerns, 8–9
Vitamin E
    cognitive function, 60
    eye health, 28–29, 308
    REACT study, 30
    VECAT study, 30
Vitamins (general), 3, 61
Volunteerism, 134

W

Waite studies, 96
Wales
    dementia, 161
    family support, 97
    fertility rates, 87
    marriage rates, 87, 89
    mortality and temperature, 104
Walker studies, 3, 127 136
Walking
    amount necessary, 8, 19
    exertion, 20
    minimum income for healthy living, 148–149
    slow gait, 18
Warm Front energy efficiency program
    housing role, 106
    policy implications, 112
Warm-up, exercise safety, 21
Weight maintenance, *see also* Exercise

dementia, 2
  energy intake, 10
Welfare system, policy implications, 79
Wellcome Trust funded project, 132
Weschler Adult Intelligence Scale, 57
Western European countries, 120
Wet age-related macular degeneration (wet
  AMD), 26
Whalley studies, 3, 51–63
Whitehall Study, 70–78
Wilkinson studies, 3, 69, 103–113, 139–151
Wilson studies, 35–49

Woods and McKiernan studies, 36
Woodward and Kawachi studies, 68
Work, 118–120, *see also* Occupation
Work ability, 157

Z

Zeaxanthein, 28–29, 31
Zinc, 28–30